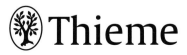

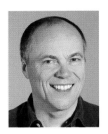

Dr. oec. troph. Karl von Koerber is leader of the Working Group on Sustainable Nutrition at the Technische Universität München, Germany. In addition, he directs the Consulting Agency for Nutrition Ecology in Munich. In 2012, both organizations were featured by the German UNESCO Commission as an official project of the UN Decade of Education for Sustainable Development (2005–2014). He gives lectures and continuing education seminars for scientists, stakeholders, and laypersons on sustainability and eating, "Nutrition Ecology," climate protection, global food issues, organic foods, and so on. He is the author of numerous books and magazine articles and advises companies, associations, hospitals, and politicians. For more information see www.ne.wzw.tum.de, www.bfeoe.de.

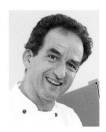

Hubert Hohler is head chef at the Buchinger Fasting Clinic at Lake Constance, Germany, where he spoils his guests with delicious wholefood fare. For more information see www.buchinger.com. In addition, he is president of Slow Food Bodensee and is a member of the network of "bio-mentors," which has been featured by the German UNESCO Commission as an official project of the UN Decade of Education for Sustainable Development (2005–2014).

We are grateful to Andreas Beier, Birgit Widhopf, Verena Kleindienst, Dr. Markus Keller, Dr. Mathias Schwarz, Dr. Anita Idel, Maike Nestle, Carmen Hübner, Thomas Schwab, Norbert Schwab, Kuno Kübler, Rosemarie Hartmann, Gunhild Schwerdtfeger, and Dorothea Heimes-Grobbel for their helpful assistance and valuable suggestions. We would also like to thank the chefs Markus Keller, Paul Rehberger, and Hubert Neidhart for their assistance with the meat and fish recipes, as well as Birgitt Ettl, Jana Heller, and the culinary team of the Buchinger Fasting Clinic for their help in the creation and analysis of the recipes. Our thanks also go to Dr. Angela Hartmann, Marie-Christine Scharf, Theresa Mühlthaler, and Anna Popp for their help with the English edition.

The Joy of Sustainable Eating

Karl von Koerber, PhD
Working Group on Sustainable Nutrition
Technische Universität München
Munich, Germany

Hubert Hohler
Head Chef
Buchinger Clinic Lake Constance
Überlingen, Germany

54 illustrations

Thieme
Stuttgart · New York

Library of Congress Cataloging-in-Publication Data
is available from the publisher.

This book is an authorized translation of the German edition published and copyrighted 2012 by TRIAS Verlag in MVS Medizinverlage Stuttgart GmbH & Co. KG, Stuttgart. Title of the German edition: Nachhaltig genießen: Rezeptbuch für unsere Zukunft.

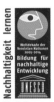

Ein Beitrag zur
Weltdekade

Translator:
Sabine Williams, Corbett, OR, USA

Photos:
Meike Bergmann, Berlin, Germany

© 2013 Georg Thieme Verlag KG,
Rüdigerstrasse 14, 70469 Stuttgart, Germany
http://www.thieme.de
Thieme Medical Publishers, Inc., 333 Seventh Avenue,
New York, NY 10001, USA
http://www.thieme.com

Cover design: Thieme Publishing Group
Typesetting by Ziegler + Müller, Kirchentellinsfurt, Germany
Printed in Germany by AZ Druck und Datentechnik GmbH, Kempten

ISBN 978-3-13-172451-9

Also available as e-book:
eISBN 978-3-13-172461-8

Table of Contents

Foreword by Alexander Mueller and Peter Glasauer (FAO)

The pleasure of eating—for all, including the generations to come

In spite of recent significant improvements in food security and nutrition outcomes worldwide, almost 870 million people continue to suffer from chronic undernourishment, and the negative health consequences of micronutrient deficiencies have continued to affect around 2 billion people in the period 2010–2012. In today's world of unprecedented technical and economic opportunities, it is entirely unacceptable that more than 100 million children under the age of five are underweight, and therefore unable to realize their full socio-economic and human potential. Childhood malnutrition is the cause of death for more than 2.5 million children every year, or nearly 7000 children every day! The right to food is a basic human right and must be realized with highest priority. No child, no woman, and no man should go to bed hungry. Additionally, the costs of hunger are huge. Hunger and malnutrition are significant obstacles to a country's economic growth and overall development.

While major efforts at many levels—including the highest political ones—are required to improve food and nutrition security worldwide, each and every consumer can participate and contribute. This book, as "simple" as it may seem, is of excellent help in this endeavor. It sensitizes and informs the reader about the issues of world hunger, and clearly shows that sustainability—a term that has gained more widespread recognition in the recent past—should not be limited to aspects of the physical environment and climate. Instead, true sustainability also means actions that are socially acceptable, culturally desirable, and economically feasible.

Laudably, the book not only motivates the reader to be part of the solution. With a collection of thoughtful, well-designed, and tempting recipes for sustainable meals it also helps to build the very skills for practicing this form of sustainability in such daily activities as eating and cooking. We congratulate the authors for this "tasteful" contribution to the issues of world hunger and its sustainable eradication.

Alexander Mueller
Assistant Director-General, Natural Resources Management and Environment Department, Food and Agriculture Organization (FAO) of the United Nations

and

Peter Glasauer, PhD
Nutrition Officer, Nutrition Division, Economic and Social Development Department, Food and Agriculture Organization (FAO) of the United Nations

Foreword by Achim Steiner (UNEP)

In the United Kingdom one of the fastest growing areas of the food market is the demand for misshapen, cosmetically challenged fruit and vegetables. In China the government has urged all organizers of large state banquets to cut unnecessary volumes of meals being prepared and a social networking initiative called "Eat Up Your Dishes" is taking the public by storm. What these and a myriad of other initiatives and actions are addressing is a growing disquiet and a determination to act on the extraordinary amount of food that is being wasted and lost across the globe.

In *developed* countries households often purchase too much food, which then goes off; supermarkets often have over-rigorous standards on the shape, appearance, and color of foods; and labeling regulations can confuse consumers about what is still edible. In *developing* countries supply chains can be fragile, power outages can trigger freezers to fail and food to spoil, and storage facilities can be prone to pests.

The loss and waste of at least one-third of the globe's food has become an emblematic example of the current unsustainable path while being an economic, ethical, and environmental challenge. Food loss and waste equate to the degradation of natural resources, from water and soils to energy and inputs like fertilizers and chemicals. Another global problem is climate change. The food sector contributes a significant proportion of greenhouse gases caused by, for example, the clearance of forests for animal feed production and methane emissions from landfills linked with food waste.

UNEP has joined forces with the Food and Agriculture Organization of the UN to catalyze scaled-up and accelerated action.

The campaign *Think–Eat–Save: Reduce Your Foodprint* is raising global awareness while bringing together fresh ideas and transformative advice.

In some countries many people believe that their own household does not waste food, though others on the same street do. Taking a look into each other's trash can be a cathartic experience.

Rediscovering the fun of cooking with leftovers, of pickling vegetables, or learning to make jam can become a family-oriented activity with a wider environmental and social purpose. Food has always been a celebration, a way of bringing people together and of sharing the tears and the joys of being human. Food is at the center of culture—in the future it will also be central to peace and security in a world of seven billion people, climbing to over nine billion in 2050.

This book, *The Joy of Sustainable Eating,* is part of a growing recognition globally and rediscovery locally of food as a precious resource worth celebrating and cherishing by everyone.

Achim Steiner
Under-Secretary-General, United Nations (UN)
and Executive Director,
United Nations Environment Programme (UNEP)

Foreword by Claus Leitzmann

The routine necessity of eating has become confusing for the consumer. In addition to the task of selecting from the excessive number of food products that has risen far beyond the 150 000 mark, numerous expectations have to be met. Specifically, one should purchase, prepare, and eat food that is in season, regionally grown, healthy, socially acceptable, economically feasible, culturally desirable, politically correct, and ecologically compatible. In addition, the diet should be balanced, not too sweet, not too high in fat, and should be eaten without leftovers. It is not surprising that consumers have difficulties in coping with this score of demands. They respond with irritation and even frustration and are discouraged from heeding any of these suggestions. This is the least favorable response that can occur and calls for action.

This book by Karl von Koerber and Hubert Hohler provides one answer to the present anxiety and confusion of the consumer because it incorporates all the well-founded recommendations. It serves as a guide to eating with pleasure and with a clear conscience. The authors recommend a rather simple way of eating, which is both prudent and enjoyable without burdening the consumer with overly detailed advice.

The book has been chosen by the UNESCO as an official contribution to the United Nations Decade of Education for Sustainable Development. Sustainability with the dimensions of health, society, environment, and economy is the basis of the recommendations in this book, a concept we introduced 35 years ago in my group for international nutrition at our university. We started with the integrated concept of "Wholesome Nutrition," followed by the new scientific discipline "Nutrition Ecology." This led to the project The New Nutrition Science, which was supported by the International Union of Nutritional Sciences, the umbrella organization for the national nutrition societies of the world, peaking in the Giessen Declaration. This concept was adopted by the World Public Health Nutrition Association. Karl von Koerber was central to this development from the beginning and has incorporated these concepts in the current book.

Food purchasing is like a ballot for the quality of our food, our health, and our future. Our current food choices will determine how coming generations will eat and live. Since we usually eat several times a day, we all have the opportunity to contribute to a better world. The recommendations and the recipes for delicious meals in this book are practical and easy to follow and they provide motivation to participate in shaping our future now.

Claus Leitzmann, PhD
Professor, Institute of Nutrition Science
University of Giessen, Germany

Foreword by Karl Ludwig Schweisfurth

Eating is our Fate

Eating is fateful
for our life, for our enjoyment of life,
for health and well-being,
depending on
whether we eat life-promoting sustenance
or cheap food products.

Eating is fateful
for our earth, for the soil
that gives us life and sustenance,
depending on how
we treat nature
with care or destructively.

Fate does not have to be inevitable.
We can take our fate
into our own hands.
We can once again change the scientific-technological
system of our agriculture and
food production
that we have set up in the last fifty years
and that is now showing us its limitations and dangers.

More and more people
eat more and more animals.
The animals of wealthy people
eat the bread/grain of poor people,
all over the world.
Together with the animals,
we are eating the earth bare.

We need a new understanding
in the way we interact with animals and with meat,
otherwise we won't be able to solve any
of the problems in the world,
not hunger and poverty,
not climate change,
not the endangered livelihoods of many farmers,
not our health problems.

All those who deal with
soil, plants, and animals and
produce food for humans
carry a heavy responsibility.
We need ethical ground rules
that tell us what we have to do and
what we may not do.
Otherwise we lack
orientation.

Karl Ludwig Schweisfurth

Master Butcher, Entrepreneur
Founder of the Schweisfurth Foundation, Munich, Germany
Founder of the Herrmannsdorfer Landwerkstätten,
Glonn near Munich, Germany
Founder of the Versuchsanstalt für Symbiotische Landwirtschaft
(Research Institute for Symbiotic Agriculture),
Glonn near Munich, Germany

Dear Readers

It gives me great pleasure to accompany you on an exciting journey to sustainability. Our book is intended to facilitate your start in this direction and to instill a desire for more—if you are not already firmly on board. It contains a wealth of background information and useful tips, as well as Hubert Hohler's delicious recipes. By putting all these together you will be able to bring more sustainability into your everyday life.

I am a scientist and initially thought that presenting the concepts of sustainability and nutrition in the first part and background information in the last part of the book would suffice as "my" guide to living sustainably. The publisher disagreed: "But Dr. von Koerber, our readers also want to know something about you personally!" And the suggestion to recount my own "path to sustainability," as it were, did prove appealing to me after all. And so it happened that two editors from the Thieme publishing house stopped by for a chat on a lovely late summer day.

Thieme: Dr. von Koerber, you are presumably one of the "most sustainable" people in Germany. Would you tell us how you became interested in nutrition and sustainability in the first place?

Dr. Karl von Koerber (KvK): Now that I think about it, I was already living more or less sustainably before the term became so popular. My parents laid the first foundation: they had their own garden where they grew organic vegetables and fruits, and they also bought organic foods in general—which was not easy and anything but normal 40 years ago.

Thieme: Nevertheless, from an organic garden it is still quite a long way to sustainability.

KvK: That's correct. I did have a key experience that proved to be a formative one in this regard. When I was 16 years old, my mother was diagnosed with cancer. She first underwent surgery in a university hospital, but the subsequent treatment failed to satisfy her health needs. A friend consequently advised her to visit a hospital for naturopathic and holistic medicine. The head physician there, Dr. Max-Otto Bruker, happened to be one of the pioneers of "Wholesome Nutrition," as well as an environmental activist. For him, diet was an important pillar of cancer therapy—and the combination of university-based and naturopathic treatments allowed my mother's condition to improve steadily. She regained her health and continued to live for a number of years in good health. Another factor that shaped me in my adolescence was the experience of attending anti-nuclear demonstrations with my parents and siblings in the 1970s. Together, we worked with the city of Marburg to get permission to install one of the first solar panel systems on the roof of my parents' house—at that time not a simple affair, even though such installations are now actively subsidized by the German government.

Thieme: As you already said, your parents were the key influence in your life. What role did your father play?

KvK: A really important one. My father's background was in agriculture, and he later worked in economics and social sciences at the universities of Giessen and Marburg. Questions that he addressed in his work were, for example, how can we improve East–West relationships or restructure the global economy, or how can we assure that the entire population on earth receives a more just income and enough to eat. Social justice was a matter of great concern to him. His last publication before he died in 1981 affected me deeply. It was titled *What Does 'Social' Mean?* He asked uncomfortable questions: for example, are people in the rich industrialized countries living at the expense of people in the developing countries? Or how does the global flow of goods function, and who earns what and where? In my early childhood I had already come into contact with all these economic and social questions addressed by my father—in combination with my mother's health-related and ecological interests.

Thieme: That does sound exciting. What happened later after high school?

KvK: While looking for a professional orientation, I found out about a course of studies in "Nutritional Science." This was a breakthrough discovery for me. I decided on the university in Giessen. Even before I began my studies, I completed an internship on an organic farm, followed by one in the kitchen of a naturopathic sanatorium with their own organic gardening operation.

Thieme: And how did this initial fascination with nutritional science develop further on?

KvK: In all honesty, it was quite quickly replaced by disillusionment. The reason for this is that my university studies were primarily dealing with vitamins and metabolism, processing technologies in the food industry, fertilizer optimization, and the origin of disease and so on. But issues such as environmental concerns, the social or ethical aspects of the production of food, organic agriculture, or holistic approaches to diet were ignored. Just imagine this: I arrived at the university as a young person, full of questions and ideas, with my first notions about where and why things might not be running smoothly in the world—and didn't receive any satisfying answers.

Thieme: I bet this was quite difficult. Did you not have any allies?

KvK: I did! In my second semester, I met Thomas Maennle. Our connection and joint efforts have by now lasted for almost four decades. Over time, other students with similar mindsets also joined us. Together, we founded the student working group "Alternative Nutrition" ("Alternative Ernährung") and this represented the turning point in the advancement of our interests.

Thieme: What exactly was the task of this study group?

KvK: We worked on topics that we found lacking in our university studies—it was like a sort of self-help group. When I think back to this time, I become quite sentimental. We studied all the alternative systems of diet and nutrition out there, from vegetarianism to dietary therapy according to Chinese medicine. We invited experts and discussed their approaches.

Thieme: This sounds quite theoretical.

KvK: No, the theory was only one aspect. In addition, we always prepared meals in accordance with each recommendation. At that time, health food stores didn't exist, and we had to be creative to find all the necessary ingredients. As a result, we started the first "Food Coop Giessen" and purchased directly from organic farmers or organic companies. In my dorm room, for instance, I may have stored a sack of grain under the bed, while Thomas kept nuts and nut butters. And after exchanges of information and discussion, we greatly enjoyed eating our home-cooked meals. Can you think of a nicer connection between theory and practice?

Thieme: Sounds wonderful! And did you then also go out to study practical applications in a larger sense?

KvK: Yes, we visited, for example, clinics, companies, or farms involved in organic agriculture. What became our personal favorite was the "Wholesome Nutrition" according to Prof. Werner Kollath, at the time represented by Dr. Bruker. Together, Thomas Maennle and I completed an internship with Dr. Bruker, which involved working in the kitchen and instruction in nutritional counseling.

Thieme: It seems that the university was less important for your professional development?

KvK: That could have easily been the case if it hadn't been for Dr. Claus Leitzmann, who came to Giessen University as a research fellow at this time. His field was called "Nutrition in Developing Countries."

Thieme: I see, social justice is coming back into play again.

KvK: Exactly. I got to know Dr. Leitzmann more closely when I participated as a research subject in a metabolism study that he directed. There, I also reported on my recent experiences with "Wholesome Nutrition" during my internship—and Dr. Leitzmann showed great interest in these holistic approaches. Our discussions, in fact, culminated in a visit with Thomas Maennle to Dr. Bruker's naturopathic clinic in Lahnstein, where we exchanged ideas.

Thieme: You also wrote a book on the topic of "Wholesome Nutrition" with Thomas Maennle and Professor Leitzmann, right?

KvK: Yes. But first, the next step was our diploma theses, which we wrote under his guidance. After their completion, we wanted to revise them for publication—and Dr. Leitzmann, recently having been appointed Professor, was willing to contribute to this book as an author. We wanted to serve as bridge builders between the naturopathic approaches and mainstream nutritional science.

Thieme: The subsequent book, published in German by Thieme/Haug, has been reprinted 11 times by now. You are therefore one of the pioneers of "Wholesome Nutrition" in Germany.

KvK: Well, I do think that the book has established itself as a standard reference in Germany over these three decades, especially because we also included demands for environmental and social sustainability. But it was not accepted with open arms everywhere. From the field of nutritional science, we received warnings: "Why don't you just stick to nutrition and stop spreading your ideology and worldview!" A completely different response came from students, nutritional counselors, physicians, teachers, and course leaders.

Thieme: And what happened during this time with your student working group in Giessen?

KvK: A number of other working groups had formed over the years. The demand by students for more connections to the ecological, social, and economic aspects in their course work continued to grow. In addition, students from other universities transferred to Giessen because our activities there had become known.

Thieme: And did these students see their expectations fulfilled?

KvK: By this time, the students were demanding the establishment of a separate professorship. Professor Leitzmann provided crucial support and coined the term "Nutrition Ecology" (*Ernährungsökologie*) for the new field. At last, the university and the government of the state of Hessen approved a new professorship.

Thieme: And everything was smooth sailing from then on.

KvK: Unfortunately not. Even though Germany's reunification was a wonderful event, it initially resulted in a rough setback for us. The government decided in 1989 to redirect any available resources in science to East German universities—this meant the end for our planned professorship at the last minute.

Thieme: What happened then, what did you do?

KvK: We enjoyed at least a partial success because the newly founded working group "Nutrition Ecology" around Professor Leitzmann at least received an additional half-time position for a research fellow. This became my first appointment after the completion of my PhD, and for about 9 years I was deeply involved in its development.

Thieme: These days you are based in Munich with your work on sustainability. How did you get there?

KvK: In 1997, I moved to southern Germany, where there was a lot of development work to be done as well. First, I founded the "Consulting Agency for Nutrition Ecology" (Beratungsbüro für ErnährungsÖkologie) and gave numerous presentations, held lecturer positions at several colleges, published professional papers, and provided consultations for businesses and associations in the German-speaking world.

Thieme: But in the meantime you are also working at a university again.

KvK: Yes, in 1998 the Technische Universität München invited me to present a lecture on "Nutrition Ecology," which received great feedback. During the last 15 years of sustained efforts, with the engaged support from students and professors, I was able to establish a range of courses that are enjoying rapidly growing popularity among students from various disciplines. For the past five years, we have been building a formal Working Group called "Sustainable Nutrition," which has so far been financed by donations from foundations, businesses, and associations. More and more students also want to write their bachelor's or master's theses with us—to the point where we are no longer able to keep up with the enormous demand.

Thieme: And are you also active on the outside, in science, education, or politics?

KvK: Of course! Today, "sustainability" is after all no longer a topic of concern to only a few individuals, but has become a guiding principle in politics and has also been accepted on supermarket shelves. Our problems have become so serious on the global level that they can only be solved by interconnected thinking and global, multigenerational activity. As a result, requests for continuing education and lectures outside the university continue to increase—especially since within the ongoing UN "Decade of Education for Sustainable Development" the year 2012 has been designated as focusing on "Sustainable Nutrition"! In this context, we are involved in numerous educational programs in schools, colleges, environmental centers, and so on, as well as in comprehensive campaigns. Fortunately, we have meanwhile been allocated the status of official project of this "Decade of Education for Sustainable Development" by the German UNESCO Commission.

Thieme: How do you succeed on a personal level in framing your life more in a direction towards sustainability?

KvK: Oh, I have lots of ideas in that regard. I have never owned my own car—we got rid of the car that we used to co-own in our previous housing community more than 20 years ago. Instead I get around by rail and bus or by bike. Sometimes I even commute a full 40 km to work in Freising—with a wonderful new electric bicycle. In addition, I generate my own eco-energy by contributing financially to wind and solar power installations. And in the area of diet, I, of course, implement the basic rules we've established that you will learn more about in this book.

Thieme: And apparently we are sitting here in a very special space.

KvK: Yes, lastly I have also concerned myself with another important topic, namely living arrangements. I have therefore intentionally moved to the new co-operative housing community "wagnis" ("venture") in East Munich, which likewise follows the requirements of sustainability. All the houses are built either according to low energy or ultra-low *passive house* standards, including terrific thermal insulation, solar systems on the roofs, eco-energy, and geothermal heat pump systems. And we have young and old, families and singles, disabled and nondisabled persons, and people from a wide variety of origins and nations, all living together—with ample communal space for various purposes—and everything is organized according to self-organizing structures that promote good neighborly relations.

Thieme: To return to our book: when the publisher approached you with the idea of writing this guide together with Hubert Hohler, you said that you knew each other well—how so?

KvK: I already knew about the Buchinger Fasting Clinic and the fact that they were practicing the dietary concepts we developed in Giessen. And ever since partaking in one of their fasting programs—which also, by the way, played a role in my decision to move to Munich—I have frequently been invited there as a lecturer at nutritional seminars for the house guests. In addition, I teach continuing education courses for the staff, sometimes also for the head chef, Hubert Hohler, and his culinary team. In this field, he is the practitioner of the two of us—for this reason the recipes in this book are obviously created by him.

Thieme: We think it is wonderful that you are basically doing exactly the same thing as you did long ago with your student working group at the university in Giessen. You connect theory with practice and motivate others to do the same.

KvK: Yes, in culinary terms! Hubert Hohler and I really hope to demonstrate that sustainability and enjoyment are not mutually exclusive. Sustainability also means true and lasting *joie de vivre*—and in the area of nutrition, also the notion of a culinary culture. If we succeed in stimulating the same desire for sustainability in our readers that we often experience in our students, participants in seminars, or professionals in culinary training, we will be overjoyed!

Thieme: Even with all this fun you are also a highly conscientious person, and the transparency of your factual statements is of great importance to you.

KvK: Yes. You will notice when reading the book that the informational parts include notes with information on sources. For a very good reason: sustainability is also concerned with fair social interactions. For me as a scientist, it therefore goes without saying that credit is given to the people or institutions to whose research we refer. A piece of sustainability within the book, you could say.

Thieme: Both Mr. Hohler and Thieme Publishers recognized the potential of your book for the international market and therefore encouraged you to consider the publication of an international edition in English. What do you see as the greatest strengths of your publication or, shall we say, that special something in comparison with similar books on this topic in English that are already available on the market?

KvK: What is special and innovative about our book is the connection between science and its practical application. Or in other words the implementation of scientific discoveries in the field of Sustainable Eating in the form of delicious recipes that are created on the basis of health-promoting, ecological, economic, and social criteria. And best of all: you then get to just enjoy and savor the meals you have prepared, without having to think of all these demands. As the title says: "The Joy of Sustainable Eating"!

Of course we are particularly delighted that not only the German edition but also the present English edition of our book has been recognized by UNESCO as "contribution for the United Nations Decade of Education for Sustainable Development." This also means that we can use the UNESCO logo on our title page.

And now I hope that all our readers will find much pleasure in reading the following introduction and the in-depth background information at the end of the book—as well as, of course, in the practical preparation and enjoyment of the delicious recipes, "sustainably" created by Hubert Hohler.

Karl von Koerber

Preface

Dear Readers,

I am delighted with the title of this book—The Joy of Sustainable Eating. It illustrates that conscious, sustainable eating and enjoyment are not mutually exclusive, but go together superbly. I live this idea every working day in my kitchen and am thrilled to share it with you through the recipes in this book.

Since my early school days I had the desire to become a cook. As a youngster I had to help out frequently in our vegetable fields. When I reached fifth grade it became my job to cultivate and harvest our asparagus plantation. That was an early morning duty before it was time to get ready for school. Naturally, that was not always a source of joy…but it taught me to appreciate fresh, home-grown foods. I became increasingly interested in the pleasures that can be created using delicious vegetables. Much to my parents' dismay, I decided that higher education was not necessary to work as a cook. When I was 15, I began my educational journey to become a chef.

In 1985, as part of my craftsman certification, I introduced wholegrain strudel dough. That was regarded as a complete "no go" by the world of haute cuisine and almost came at the price of my award. As you can see, even back then I was dedicated to a healthy diet. I was certainly influenced by the fact that my father had suffered two heart attacks by this time and he was only in his mid-forties. My eating and cooking habits had caused me various health problems as well: I was overweight and had elevated blood pressure and cholesterol levels. The experiences surrounding my father's health issues gradually caused a change of heart and the health aspects of food preparation became even more important to me. After passing the craftsman's examination, I continued my education with additional training and certifications as dietary cook and gourmet chef for "Wholesome Nutrition."

Since 1997, I have been Chef de Cuisine at the Buchinger Fasting Clinic at Lake Constance in Germany. My daily work is guided by the idea of using healthy, Fair Trade foods and preparing them in a resource-efficient way. My dishes are meant to demonstrate that health and enjoyment are not contradictory, but can go hand in hand.

I prefer internationally influenced cuisine. My cooking is inspired by Mediterranean as well as by Oriental dishes. There is only one requirement—the foods I use must be 100% organic and seasonal. Processed foods do not make their way into my pots and pans.

For the past few years, the Slow Food organization has become close to my heart. Slow Food is a global nonprofit organization that believes "that everyone has a fundamental right to the pleasure of good food and consequently the responsibility to protect the heritage of food, tradition and culture that make this pleasure possible." Today, there are more than 60 regional Slow Food groups in Germany, one of which I have headed since 2007 at Lake Constance. Our motto is: "Preserve enjoyment, diversity of species, and true natural flavors!" We support responsible and appropriate agriculture and fishing, as well as traditional food production. In this context, it is of utmost importance to us to promote and facilitate contact and communication between producers, merchants, and consumers. It is crucial for people to know and understand where their food is coming from, how it is handled, and how to recognize fresh quality foods. Sustainability plays a vital part in these considerations.

In addition to my involvement with Slow Food, I have been a member of BioMentoren since 2009. BioMentoren is a network of restaurant proprietors, operations managers, chefs de cuisine, and purchasers. Each BioMentoren business member holds the organic food certification and uses species-appropriate husbandry, Fair Trade, and sustainable fishing products. In 2012, the BioMentoren project was awarded the UNESCO title "Official Project of the United Nations Decade of Education for Sustainable Development." We are very proud of this recognition. It confirms that we are on the right track to get our message across.

For now, I wish you joy and success while trying out my recipes. It is my goal to introduce recipes that are healthy and tasty, and especially easy to follow.

Hubert Hohler

Conversion Table

Weight

Metric	English (U. S.)
1 milligram (mg)	0.002 grain (0.000 035 ounce [oz])
1 gram (g) (1000 mg)	0.04 oz
1 kilogram (kg) (1000 g)	35.27 oz (2.20 pound [lb])

English (U. S.)	Metric
1 grain	64.80 mg
1 oz	28.35 g
1 lb	453.60 g (0.45 kg)

Volume

Metric	English (U. S.)
1 milliliter (mL)	0.03 oz
1 liter (L) (1000 mL)	2.12 pint (pt)
1 L	1.06 quart (qt)
1 L	0.27 gallon (gal)

English (U. S.)	Metric
1 fluid ounce (fl o)	30 mL
1 pt	470 mL
1 qt	950 mL
1 gal	3.79 L

Liquids

Metric	English (U. S.)
1 mL	$^1/_5$ teaspoon (tsp)
5 mL	1 tsp
15 mL	1 tablespoon (tbsp)
30 mL	$^1/_8$ cup
60 mL	$^1/_4$ cup
100 mL (1 deciliter [dl])	$^2/_5$ cup (approx.)
120 mL	$^1/_2$ cup
240 mL	1 cup
480 mL	1 pt

Length

Metric	English (U. S.)
1 centimeter (cm)	0.3937 inch (in)
5 cm	1.9685 in
10 cm	3.9370 in
50 cm	19.6850 in
1 meter (m)	39.37 008 in (1.09 yards [yd])
30 m	98.4252 feet (ft) (32.80 yd)
50 m	164.04 199 ft (54.68 yd)
100 m	109.36 yd (0.062 mi)
1 kilometer (km) (1000 m)	0.62 mile (mi)
50 km	31.06 mi

English (U. S.)	Metric
1 in	2.54 cm
5 in	12.7 cm
12 in (1 ft)	30.48 cm
15 in	38.1 cm
36 in (3 ft; 1 yd)	91.44 cm
1 ft (12 in)	30.48 cm
50 ft	15.24 m
1 mi	1.61 km

Temperature	
Celsius	**Fahrenheit**
1 °C	33.8 °F
5 °C	41 °F
20 °C	68 °F
50 °C	122 °F
100 °C (water boils)	212 °F
180 °C (moderate oven)	356 °F
200 °C	392 °F
220 °C	428 °F
250 °C	482 °F
Fahrenheit	**Celsius**
32 °F (water freezes)	0 °C
60 °F	15 °C
70 °C	21 °C
100 °F	37.7 °C
200 °F	93.3 °C
212 °F (water boils)	100 °C
300 °F	148.8 °C
350 °F (moderate oven)	175 °C
400 °F	204.4 °C
500 °F (extremely hot oven)	260 °C

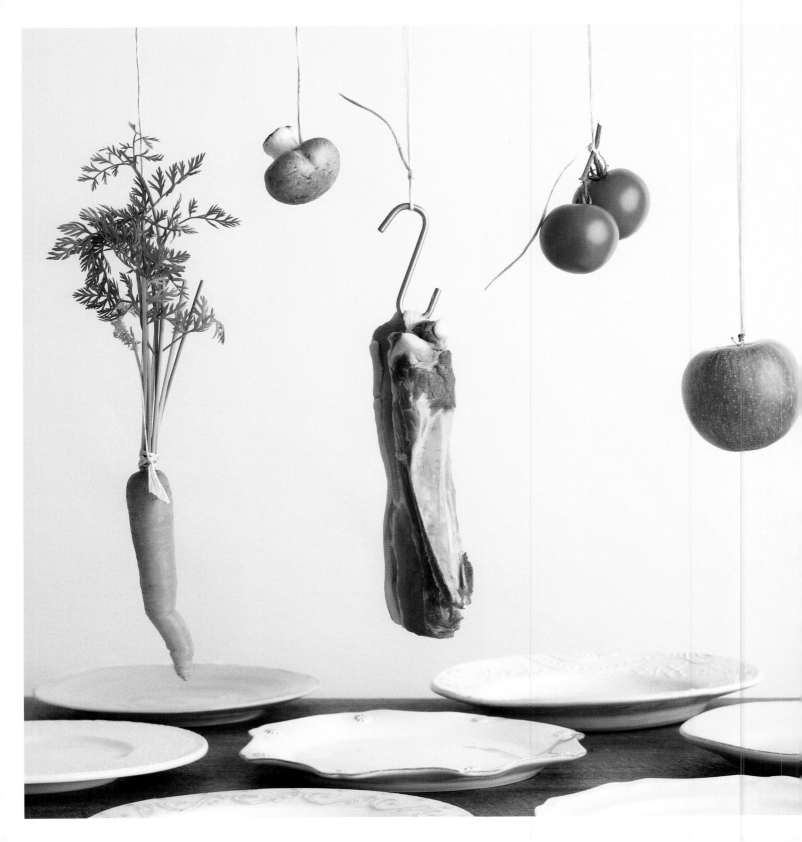

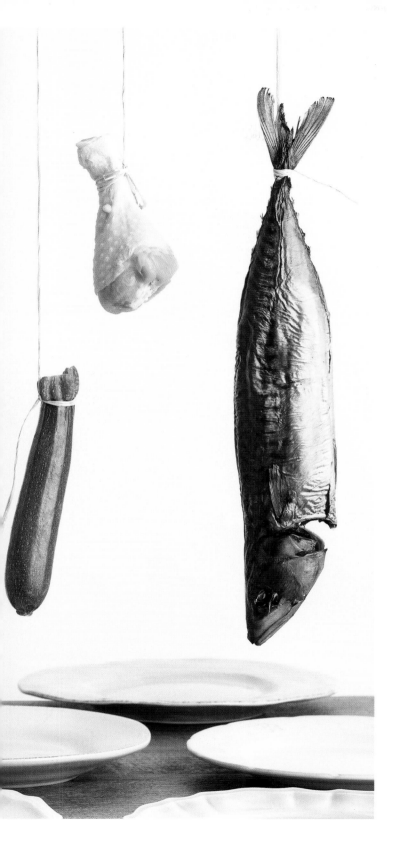

Why It's Worth Eating Sustainably

Do you often find yourself standing in front of a supermarket shelf and wondering what you can still buy without hesitation? You want to shop more consciously, eat sustainably, but you still feel unsure? This book will tell you why organic food is a viable alternative and how you can make a sustainable diet a reality without missing out on the joy of eating.

The Four Dimensions of Sustainability in Eating

If we were still eating today as our grandparents once did, animals in agricultural production would certainly be raised under more species-appropriate conditions. Meat, fish, and eggs would not be eaten daily but would be a rare luxury. In those days, you would only see a roast on the table on Sunday. Cake made with lots of eggs was a weekend treat. Vegetables and fruit were either grown in the garden or came from the local area.

Nobody would have imagined then that it would be possible some day to buy cheap tomatoes all year long. In many cases, these tomatoes are grown and harvested by immigrants from developing countries under questionable working conditions. Cultivating tomatoes in huge plantations consumes so much water that the local groundwater level drops precipitously, resulting in water shortages.

Nowadays we eat food whose history we are rarely familiar with—often, we know little about its production, processing, and origin, or retail and transport. Its ingredients or additives are largely unknown to us. We consume too many animal-based foods—and too many heavily processed products whose valuable ingredients have often been destroyed. It is becoming rare for us to prepare our meals ourselves, and cooking is increasingly being relegated to the sidelines for our spare time. The products we consume are often prepared in advance, extravagantly packaged, and in many cases frozen. Then we often heat them up in the microwave or eat them cold, straight out of the package. Less and less frequently,

we turn to actual foodstuff; instead, we increasingly choose products that are advertised in terms of "wellness," "anti-aging," or "probiotic."[1]

What and how much we eat has significant consequences for our body, as well as for the natural environment, for other people, and for the economic

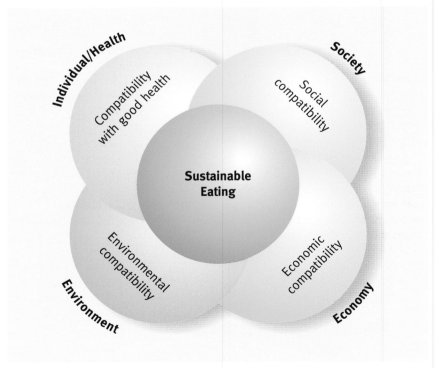

▲ The four dimensions of sustainable eating.[2]

2

situation of everybody involved. In this context, we speak of the four dimensions of a sustainable lifestyle: health, environment, society, and economy (see illustration). Our choice of food has both regional and global effects. The three dimensions of environment, society, and economy are summarized under the political model of "sustainability," on which the 178 member states reached a worldwide consensus at the UN Conference on Environment and Development in Rio de Janeiro in 1992. In the context of diet, health has been added as the fourth dimension.[1,2]

Sustainability refers to a global development that aims at satisfying the needs of present generations without jeopardizing the ability of future generations to satisfy *their* needs—as well as the notion that the populations of the industrialized countries should no longer live at the expense of the populations of the so-called developing (poor) countries. The goal is to create equality of opportunity for all humans living on earth today while at the same time securing the same for future generations. Let us now take a closer look at the interconnections between the four dimensions of sustainability (for sources and more detailed information on these concepts, see the two German publications von Koerber and Kretschmer[1] and von Koerber, Männle, and Leitzmann[2]).

In Harmony with the Environment

All too often we humans strain the environment and thereby the natural foundations of life beyond their limit—most notably by our extravagant lifestyle in industrialized countries. This frequently occurs at the expense of the environment:

- Pollution of air, water, soil, and food with harmful chemicals
- More greenhouse gases in the atmosphere and rising temperatures
- Global climate change: melting glaciers and polar ice, storms, droughts, forest fires, flooding of rivers, rising sea levels, etc.
- Destruction of the ozone layer ("ozone hole")
- Soil loss from erosion, compaction, salinization, etc.
- Dying forests (*Waldsterben*) and logging, for example to create arable land for the cultivation of soy beans as animal fodder
- Changes in the cultural landscape, for example the disappearance of hedges
- Declining biodiversity in both plants and animals
- Overfishing in the oceans
- Water shortages in many areas of the world

Important: You can contribute to the preservation of the environment and of natural resources—among other actions also by the way you eat.

Fair Prices—Fair Wages

Many people earn their living by producing, processing, transporting, preparing, retailing, informing about, or advertising food for other people. In many highly industrialized countries, the food sector is one of the most important branches of the economy, which is, however, engaged in often ruinous competition. Due to falling food prices, many farmers, but also processing companies and retailers, are no longer able to cover their costs. Take milk prices as an example—they have been falling for so long that dairy farmers do not get paid enough per liter. Prices no longer honestly reflect the costs involved in real-life production; they include neither the ecological nor the social follow-up costs.

On a global scale, many people in developing countries receive inadequate wages for their work and are therefore simply too poor to buy enough food for themselves, even though enough food is being produced.

Important: Fair prices for farmers worldwide pave the way for the protection of their income and preserve and create jobs.

Social Cooperation for All—Worldwide

More than a third of the global grain harvest is fed to livestock in order to produce meat, milk, and eggs.[3] The main problem with this situation is that in many cases the conversion of plant-based products, which humans would for the most part be able to consume directly, into animal products is not very efficient. To produce 1 kg of meat (see conversion table on pp. XVIII – XIX), for example, many times this weight is needed in grain, which could just be eaten directly in the form of bread. Approximately 70 to 90 % of dietary calories can be wasted as so-called refinement loss.[4] In light of the fact that there are almost a billion undernourished people in the world, this is a great waste of raw materials.[5] Ruminant animals like cattle, sheep, and goats, however, are not dependent on grain or soy. They are able to convert grass, a resource that is not utilizable by humans, into high-grade food. When they graze on grass out in pasture they do not compete with humans for food (see pp. 113 and 114).

Many of our consumer products, like coffee, tea, chocolate, and bananas, are produced in developing countries under often inhumane living and working conditions. Especially the different forms of child labor, defined as "exploitative," are no longer ethically tenable. A good alternative are Fair Trade–certified products (p. 128).

But even in many "First World" countries, agriculture is plagued by social problems: many operations have already been forced out of business, especially because the profit margin from the sale of agricultural products is too small.

Important: When you buy fewer animal products and more Fair Trade foods, you contribute to better living and working conditions worldwide.

Our Own Rewards: Health and Enjoyment

From a global perspective the state of human health has two faces. In poor countries in the "Global South" malnutrition predominates as a result of poverty and lack of food. Every day, roughly 21 000 children under the age of 5 lose their lives, a third up to half as the result of malnutrition.[6]

In wealthy, industrialized countries, on the other hand, health problems are frequently related to sedentary lifestyles, overeating, stress, smoking, and high alcohol consumption. Diet-related diseases that are the result of an excessive, inadequate, or unbalanced diet include dental caries, excess weight, type 2 diabetes, high blood pressure, cardiovascular disorders, gout, sluggish intestines, etc. These so-called "prosperity diseases" are now on the rise among the wealthier classes of many developing countries.

Important: Generous amounts of fresh vegetables and fruit and in general a primarily plant-based diet with sparingly processed foods keeps you healthy and is tasty.

MOTTO

The motto of sustainable eating: Eating with enjoyment and responsibility—for all humans on earth and for future generations.

The Food Groups

The following information on the food groups is based on a German book on "Wholesome Nutrition" by von Koerber, Männle, and Leitzmann.[2]

Vegetables and Fruits: Crunchy and Fresh to the Table

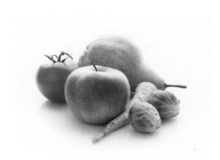

We all know the saying: "An apple a day keeps the doctor away." This suggests the key role that fresh fruits and vegetables play in our diet.

Important Nutrients

You are already eating plenty of vegetables and fruits? Wonderful! In that case you are supplying your body with lots of vitamins, minerals, dietary fiber, and phytochemicals (e.g., sulfides or glucosinolates). The high nutrient density of beets, pumpkins, etc., and their low energy content play an important role in lowering the risks of

becoming overweight, developing high blood pressure, cardiovascular disease, and various cancers. If you only eat one or two portions of vegetables and fruits a day you can find many suggestions for more vegetarian meals in the recipe section of this book. As a rule of thumb, the share of vegetables should be greater than that of fruits.

We recommend eating vegetables and fruits both cooked and raw (as fresh food). Many vitamins and phytochemicals are heat-sensitive and can be destroyed; in other cases, for example beta-carotenes in carrots, heating them improves their absorption. Most types of vegetables and fruits are very enjoyable when eaten raw—chopped in a salad or by taking a bite directly. Even broccoli tastes wonderful when grated raw as a salad—try the Broccoli, Pear, and Cashew Salad that you can find on page 38. Exceptions, however, are green beans and other legumes, as well as potatoes, which must be cooked to render unwanted ingredients harmless.

When you stew or steam vegetables gently, many important nutrients are preserved.

Fresh, Ripe, Local, and Seasonal

Locally grown, seasonal fresh vegetables and fruits are particularly recommended (p. 120). Because they are able to ripen fully before they are sold, they taste so delicious and contain more valuable ingredients. Vegetables and fruits that are out of season, as well as exotic fruits like mango, papaya, and pineapple, on the other hand, are often transported from far-away countries and are extravagantly packaged. This is costly in terms of money and energy and is damaging to the climate, especially when imported products are delivered by plane.[7] Before going shopping, it is worth considering which produce is in season to avoid products from heated greenhouses.

Cooling frozen vegetables and fruits also consumes a lot of energy—in the form of electricity. Likewise, the production of ready-made meals and of preserved vegetables and fruits in cans and glass jars is a very energy-intensive process. In addition, this type of processing degrades many important nutrients. Nevertheless, it is still better to resort to canned tomatoes and similar products in winter than to buy highly energy-intensive greenhouse products or goods that have been transported by truck or even plane over several thousand kilometers.

Note: Always wash or scrub fresh vegetables and fruits carefully because they can be contaminated, especially on the surface, with heavy metals or, in conventional cultivation, with pesticides.

TIP

Savor the great diversity of vegetables and fruits—a large proportion of them raw and unheated. Look forward to fresh local vegetables from your area that were harvested ripe.

buckwheat, you should try the Buckwheat and Oat Burgers (p. 74) or the Buckwheat Sauerkraut Casserole (p. 62) in the recipe section.

The Darker the Healthier: Wholegrain Is Best

Cereals contain an abundance of carbohydrates, proteins, vitamins, minerals, phytochemicals (e.g., polyphenols and saponins), and dietary fiber. To fully enjoy the health benefits of these ingredients, however, it is best to choose whole grains. This form contains the maximum amount of all the above-mentioned nutrients since they are found primarily in the surface layers and germ buds of the grain (p. 123). Wholegrain products and prepared foods like bread, rolls, flakes, cereal germ, muesli, noodles, casseroles, burgers, or just natural brown rice all play a role in protecting us against cardiovascular diseases, cancer, and type 2 diabetes.

With the exception of wholegrain flour, store-bought flour carries a type number in some European countries, for example, in Germany and in France. The higher the type number, the higher the nutrient content and therefore the darker the color. Light-colored types of flour, so-called superfine or cake flour, generally have a low type number. In this form there are only few nutrients from the surface layers and germ buds left. This same rule also applies to foods made from light-colored flours, such as white bread, some rye breads, white

Cereals: A Grainy Treat

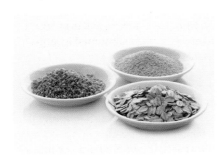

Whether in the form of bread, muesli, pancakes, or casseroles: cereals are an extremely versatile staple food that provides us with energy and many vital nutrients. Do yourself a favor and choose whole grains that were grown organically.

The Rich Diversity of Grain

The seven cereals wheat, rye, oats, barley, rice, maize, and millet form the most important major food sources in the world. In addition, we have the earliest cultivated forms of wheat, including spelt, einkorn, and khorasan wheat (also known by its trade name of Kamut). Green spelt grain is a form of spelt that is harvested half ripe and then dried. Lastly, we can explore buckwheat, quinoa, and amaranth, which strictly speaking should not be included among the cereals. Being plant seeds, we can nevertheless use them like a cereal. Because they do not contain gluten they are a good alternative for people with celiac disease who are intolerant to this protein. If you have, for example, never cooked with toast, light-colored pastries, white noodles, cornflakes—as well as white rice. In the United States and United Kingdom there is no such numbering system, but the various types of flour can be distinguished by the nutritional facts given on the packages.

To preserve the nutrients contained in grain it is best to process it as gently as possible: crushed and soaked, rolled freshly into flakes or even germinated in fresh grain muesli; cooked as a side dish, burgers, or casserole; or as flour for cooking and baking. To prevent the formation of the harmful substance acrylamide, avoid excessive browning during baking or frying.

Tip

Grind your grain fresh, right before baking or cooking. In many health food stores you can find grain mills that you can use to grind or crush whole grains right there.

the climate. Instant mixes for mashed potatoes, potato dumplings, or potato pancakes have lost many of the great health benefits of potatoes due to the numerous processing steps, but particularly the intensive drying at high temperatures. They also require a lot of energy to manufacture.

Storing Them in a Cool, Dry, and Dark Place

Potatoes are members of the nightshade (*Solanaceae*) family and should therefore be stored cool, dry, and dark. If they show green spots or begin to sprout they have been exposed to light. These parts should be cut out liberally—they contain relatively high levels of solanine, which can lead to headaches, vomiting, or diarrhea, and even worse symptoms when consumed in larger quantities.

The Inexhaustible Diversity of Potatoes

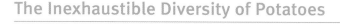

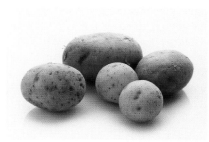

Potatoes—we eat them boiled, peeled or unpeeled, in potato salad, in soups and stews, blended into mashed potatoes or potato dumplings, roasted, grilled, or deep-fried (French fries). The diversity of varieties and methods of preparation are practically unlimited.

Ideally Pure and Not Heavily Processed

Potatoes contain mostly carbohydrates, and in addition many important protein building blocks (amino acids),

vitamins C, B$_1$, and niacin, and the minerals magnesium and potassium. Nevertheless, many nutrients get lost during processing. The more potatoes are processed, the higher the loss of nutrients. Your healthiest choice is boiled unpeeled potatoes, since boiling them in the peel preserves the original valuable nutrients (p. 126). In addition, these are then easily processed further into, for example, mashed potatoes or potato dumplings. If you peel potatoes before boiling them, many nutrients are lost by leaching into the water.

Potato chips and French fries contain a lot of fat and salt. Chips have flavoring agents added to give them the desired taste but provide hardly any important nutrients. Deep-frying, however, can produce harmful substances such as acrylamide. On top of this, their production, storage, and packaging require a lot of energy, which is detrimental to

Tip

By buying your potatoes locally, you at the same time support the farmers, for whom potatoes may be an important source of income. By shortening transport distances we are able to protect the climate and the environment. Some organic growers have returned to cultivating traditional varieties like purple potatoes (a very old, South American variety) or Russian fingerlings, for example.

Give Peas a Chance! Legumes Have a Lot to Offer

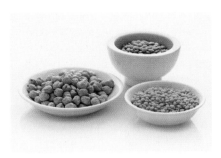

Legumes appear on our menu much too infrequently and some are almost relegated to history, and yet there are innumerable delicious varieties of lentils, peas, beans, and chickpeas.

An Abundance of Valuable Ingredients

The time has come to vindicate legumes: consuming large amounts reduces the risks of becoming overweight, developing type 2 diabetes, high blood pressure, and coronary heart disease. In addition to their appealing outside, their inner value is quite impressive as well. Legumes and legume-based products such as tofu and sandwich spreads generally have a low fat content but contain a lot of valuable protein. As a result, they are a great plant-based alternative to meat, sausage, and cheese. Whether they are du Puy lentils, borlotti beans, or scarlet runner beans, they also contain, like all legumes, an abundance of complex carbohydrates, fiber, and important vitamins, minerals, and phytochemicals.

Processed products as well are now available in many delicious variations: for example, as soy milk from soy beans or as smoked or herbed tofu. Products like textured soy meat, on the other hand, are not recommended because the valuable ingredients in legumes have been damaged by the extremely heavy processing. In addition, they generally contain numerous additives and flavoring agents.

Proper Preparation of Legumes

We have to heat legumes before we can eat them because they contain a number of harmful substances in their raw state. In addition, they contain so-called oligosaccharides. These indigestible carbohydrates are responsible for the flatulence often experienced after eating legumes. Once you start eating legumes more frequently, however, your intestinal flora gradually gets used to them. With the exception of lentils, legumes should be soaked overnight or for at least 4 hours. This reduces the cooking time and increases their digestibility. It is best to cook legumes in their soaking liquid. Herbs and spices can go in the pot, but salt and vinegar or lemon juice should only be added at the end because otherwise legumes will not become tender. And that is one of the key points here: legumes should be cooked until they are soft, not just "al dente." Ideally, legumes should be allowed to rest for 30 minutes in cook-

ing water after cooking until tender. To increase digestibility you can prepare them with herbs and spices from the umbelliferous and labiate families, such as savory, fennel, marjoram, or caraway. You can find a summery salad, Du Puy Lentils and Radicchio, on page 36. And whenever you cook legumes, always cook a little extra because they store well for a few days in the refrigerator.

Tip

Lentils, peas, beans, chickpeas, and so on are extremely inexpensive, store well without refrigeration, and are available all year long. Best if they are organic and locally grown!

Nuts, Oilseeds, and Oily Fruits: Small but Mighty

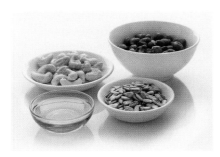

Nuts and oilseeds offer healthy, crunchy fun and improve mueslis, salads, breads, and other baked goods. Their season starts in the fall, and for the holidays at the latest you will find them on plates of assorted holiday treats or in fruit cake.

Small Power Packs

Sunflower and pumpkin seeds, sesame and flax seeds are all considered oilseeds, while oily fruits include, for example, olives and avocados. As a source of important nutrients like vital fatty acids, protein, vitamins, minerals, fiber, and phytochemicals, nuts and oilseeds help to improve our health. Their nutritional composition with mono- and polyunsaturated fatty acids is so ideal that we can use them, for example, to lower cholesterol levels and prevent cardiovascular disease. Nuts and oilseeds are particularly beneficial when eaten raw. They are also delicious when roasted but it is best not to leave them in the hot pan for too long as harmful substances like acrylamide can form.

Nuts, oilseeds, and oily fruits are, however, relatively high in fat and you should therefore enjoy them regularly in all their diversity but in moderation. Even though they are quite filling, when you enjoy too much of them your scales will let you know!

Nuts and oilseeds are also sold salted or sweetened (candied), but the high salt or sugar content of these products is problematic. Children especially are known to love chocolate-nut spreads, but these contain so much sugar that nut butters, for example, from hazelnuts or almonds, are a better alternative. You can get chocolate-nut spreads in health food stores that are sweetened with less sugar or with unrefined cane sugar or honey (p. 15). On page 25 you can find a recipe for home-made chocolate spread.

Storing Them Properly and Not Too Long

When nuts are stored incorrectly they can grow mold or become rancid. It is therefore better not to buy fresh nuts and oilseeds in large amounts—ideally buy them still in the shell so you can crack them yourself—and to store them cool and dry and not for too long. In the fall you can buy fresh walnuts or hazelnuts as well as sunflower and pumpkin seeds at farmers' markets—here it is worth asking for local products. However, even nuts that may be imported

from far away (e.g., cashews, Brazil nuts, or macadamia nuts) are fine to enjoy now and then as a special treat—as long as they are Fair Trade and organically grown. Try the Fennel Zucchini Lasagne with Cashew Nut Sauce on page 68. A wonderful dish for guests!

Tip

On walks and cycling trips in the summer keep your eyes open for wild nut trees; you can gather fresh nuts there in the fall.

More Flavor with Appropriate Fats and Oils

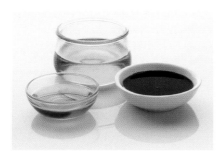

Edible fats and oils are particularly good for enhancing flavor. Because they taste so good we are often tempted to eat too much of them.

Important and Good in Moderation

Fats and oils play an important role in our diet—on bread, for cooking, for roasting, for baking, and in salads. It is, however, important to use them in moderation—about 30% of our energy supply should come from fat, which is about 60–80 g per day.[8] Our high fat consumption in industrialized countries is a contributing factor to the rise in excess weight and its secondary diseases, such as type 2 diabetes, high blood pressure, and lipometabolic disorders, and most likely increases the risk of various forms of cancer.

We can differentiate between visible fats and hidden fats. While butter on bread, for example, or olive oil in salad is visible as an ingredient, the fat content in meat, sausage, milk, cheese, and nuts or the added fat in chocolate and ready-made products is not directly apparent. Foods that naturally contain fat like meat or dairy products make up a large proportion of our daily fat supply, followed by sweets, baked goods, cooking oils, and plant-based margarines.

Variety with Canola, Olive, and Sunflower Oil

Fats and oils contain a variety of fatty acids: saturated as well as mono- and polyunsaturated. Animal-based foods in particular deliver the problematic saturated fatty acids. Our average consumption of these tends to be too high. Studies have shown that a lower consumption of saturated fatty acids and a higher consumption of mono- and polyunsaturated fatty acids has a positive effect on blood lipids. One result is, for example, that the level of unhealthy LDL-cholesterol in the blood is lowered, which in turn contributes to the protection against cardiovascular disease. To eat more vegetarian meals also means to consume less saturated fatty acids. Plant oils such as canola, olive, or sunflower oil, contain mono- and polyunsaturated fatty acids in a healthy composition. Butter and nonhydrogenated plant margarine are fine in moderation as well. Coconut oil or palm kernel oil, on the other hand, should be used only rarely because they have a high content of saturated fatty acids. We should also stay away from foods that contain the undesirable trans fatty acids, such as certain baked goods, French fries, potato chips, instant soups, ready-made meals, as well as sweets and snack foods.

Cold-pressed and Virgin

Make sure you choose cold-pressed, virgin oils instead of the more common heavily processed, extracted and refined oils (e.g., common salad oils). Cold-pressing preserves most of the valuable ingredients and flavors of the original fruits; these oils have a much stronger flavor, and they are ideally suited for mixing into dressings. Because of their naturalness they can turn rancid more quickly and should therefore be stored in the refrigerator—and not for too long. Avoid the hydrogenated fats in common margarines, as well as the products made from them. Why don't you look around in your health food store for regional oilseeds or nuts and for butters produced by local dairies! Because of their shorter transport distance they are also preferable from an ecological perspective.

Tip

Use fats and oils selectively and sparingly! Add more fresh herbs and spices to improve the flavor!

Milk: Delight from the Pasture

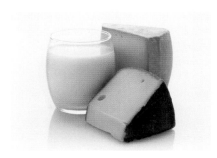

As babies our mothers' breast milk provides us with everything that we need. And even in adulthood milk remains an important food source for us.

Vital Nutrients

Milk and dairy products contain protein with a high level of essential amino acids, many important vitamins (especially B_2 and B_{12}), and minerals like calcium. Its vitamin B_{12} content makes milk a good supplement for a lacto-ovo vegetarian diet. Because of potential nutrient deficiencies (especially vitamins B_{12}, B_2, and calcium and protein) a vegan diet (a vegetarian diet that excludes meat, eggs, dairy products and all other animal-derived ingredients) is not recommended.[2] If you want to follow a vegan diet make sure that you are fully informed and take advantage of nutritional counseling. Of particular importance are high-quality plant-based sources of vitamin B_2 and calcium. Plant foods either contain little or only traces of vitamin B_{12}—for a safe vegan diet it is therefore necessary to ensure an adequate supply of this vitamin by means of enriched foods and/or supplements (which technically speaking contradicts the fundamental idea of a natural diet without chemical additives).

Don't Go Overboard with Dairy Products

Milk and dairy products are fatty foods. When cutting calories is indicated, products with low fat content might make sense. Even whole milk and cultured products (like yoghurt, sour milk, or kefir, a fermented milk drink made with kefir grains) are quite acceptable— but then only in limited quantities. In many cases, these products do contain greater amounts of fat-soluble vitamins and those substances that are responsible for the good taste. Crème fraîche, sour cream, and heavy (double) whipping cream contain a lot of fat. Normal fruit yoghurts with sugar, additives, and artificial flavors are less advisable— organic fruit yoghurts, on the other hand, are available without artificial flavors and with natural sweeteners. Buttermilk is naturally low in fat, and among cheeses those that contain less fat can also taste quite delicious.

Dairy products play an important role but should not be enjoyed in excess—it is better to choose high-quality, fair prices, and organic production (p. 116). Tasty plant-based alternatives are, for example, oat, almond, or soy milk, or the cheese-like tofu. These days, you can even find "yoghurt" or "cream" made from soy beans as well as many vegetarian spreads.

Tip

It is best to choose dairy products from animals that are raised humanely and ecologically and sustainably pastured on permanent grassland from your area. To avoid the loss of nutrients, choose pasteurized milk over ultra-high temperature (UHT) milk (as well as products made from it).
More and more research shows that untreated raw milk can protect us from allergies and asthma. Additionally it contains the greatest possible amount of vital nutrients. On the other hand, though, it harbors the risk of serious infections. We therefore recommend that raw milk should not be consumed by pregnant women, infants, small children, sick people, or people with a weakened immune system.

Meat, Fish, and Eggs: Less Is More

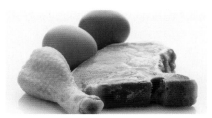

Animal-based foods contribute to our diet by supplying vital nutrients. A certain amount of meat, sausage, fish, and eggs can certainly have its place in a healthy and sustainable diet.

With Meat, Sausage, and Eggs Moderation Is in Order

The high consumption of animal-based foods common today can also contribute to diet-related disorders because they can contain a lot of dietary energy, fat, saturated fatty acids, cholesterol, and purines (p. 115). If we continue to eat such large amounts and if world-wide demand increases, global problems like world hunger, climate change, water shortages, and waste of resources will worsen (pp. 112–115). In addition, a moderate consumption of meat is easier on the wallet.

Fish: Bones of Contention

Many species of fish are high in fat but also contain essential omega-3 fatty acids. Nevertheless, it is also possible to supply these with plant-based oils like flax, hemp, rape, walnut, and soy oil. These contain alpha-linolenic acids from which our body can form omega-3 fatty acids. Deep-sea fish contributes to our intake of iodine,[9] but it can, however, be contaminated with pollutants. In spite of its health-related benefits, a diet high in fish from conventional sources is problematic in ecological and social terms.

Currently, roughly 75% of commercially utilized fish species are overfished or nearly so. Every year, moreover, many millions of tons of fish and other marine animals are caught in nets as so-called "bycatch," killed, and then thrown back into the ocean. Illegal poaching by industrial fishing fleets, but also legal fishing on the basis of EU fishing quotas and fisheries agreements, can cause local fishers, for example in African countries, to end up empty-handed. They are then threatened by unemployment, poverty, and migration. There are only a few fish species at the moment that are both ecologically and socially "acceptable." For more information regarding which kinds of fish you can enjoy without concern, see the Greenpeace and WWF web pages on the internet at www.greenpeace.org/international/en/campaigns/oceans/seafood and www.worldwildlife.org/what/globalmarkets/fishing/sustainableseafood.html.

More and more often, fish, crabs, shrimp, and so on are raised on farms by so-called aquaculture. This also includes local pond-farming by which we raise fish such as trout or carp. In conventional production, however, the number of fish is often too high, causing conditions that are not species-appropriate and at the same time polluting the water and promoting disease. This in turn results in intensive treatment with medications, which presents health and ecological risks. In addition, they are often partly fed with fish meal made from ocean fish, which again contributes to the fisheries crisis.

FACTS

Using All the Edible Parts of the Animal

In the few meat recipes found in this book the focus is on using, as much as possible, all parts of the animal, not only cutlets, chops, and fillets, but also the less valuable parts. If these are not utilized this is an unsustainable waste. The export of less valuable animal parts (which cannot be sold here) to Africa, for example, causes much damage there as this practice undercuts the prices of local producers who are then no longer able to compete and are forced out of production. The meat recipes are designed for six to 10 people because they are mostly stews that require more time in the oven, which makes the expenditure of labor and energy too high for fewer people.

Buy meat, sausage, fish, and eggs that come from organically raised and fed animals (see p. 119 for organic food signs).
Organic eggs are marked in the EU by the symbol "0" and in the United States with the USDA Organic seal and stamped 100% organic. Fish that comes from sustainable fishery and aquaculture can be identified, for example, by the MSC (Marine Stewardship Council) seal.

www.usda.gov

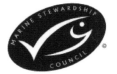

www.msc.org

Drinks: Sip by Sip to Health

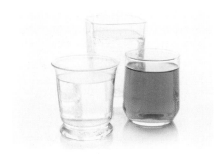

Water is indispensable to our bodily processes. It makes up roughly 60% of our body. If we do not drink regularly we suffer from fatigue, reduced productivity, or headaches.

First Choice for Drinks: Tap Water

We have to use food and drink to replace the amount of fluids that we eliminate via urine, skin, lungs, and feces. Unfortunately, we cannot rely solely on our sensation of thirst to notify us when we might need to drink more. By the time we feel thirsty our body is already suffering from slight dehydration. The key lies in drinking regularly and sufficiently throughout the course of the day, which means at least 1.5 L or more per day depending on the surrounding temperature and physical activity.[8]

To satisfy our fluid requirements we ideally recommend tap water in countries where it is controlled by rigorous standards. Bottled water is also good for our health, but—like other bottled drinks—has an unfavorable environmental record. This is due to the high energy consumption required for processing, bottling, transport, and return transport of the bottles. And it is far more expensive than the water that comes out of the tap. You do not always have to drink plain tap water either: try unsweetened herbal and fruit teas, grain coffee, and diluted fruit and vegetable juices. Undiluted juices and milk are not suitable for quenching your thirst because they are high in energy.

Coffee and Tea—Treats in Moderation

Coffee and green and black tea are not appropriate as thirst quenchers either— only in moderation as an occasional treat. They contain caffeine, which has a stimulating effect on the cardiovascular system. As a result, we get the sensation of being awake without really recharging our energy. Later on we tend to get even more tired, drink yet more coffee, and so on. High caffeine consumption can lead to sleep disorders, headaches, and stomach problems. When you do drink coffee or tea, choose Fair Trade products so that you support higher incomes for the farmers and workers and certain environmental standards in developing countries (p. 128).

Drinks that are sweetened with a lot of sugar or artificial sweeteners such as fruit nectars, juice drinks, soft drinks, energy drinks, and sports drinks are not recommended. Alcoholic drinks are considered a treat to be enjoyed in moderation and on special occasions.

In the morning, prepare herbal or fruit tea for the whole day and put it in a vacuum flask. And on hot summer days serve cool as a delicious refreshing drink.

Give Up Herbs and Spices? Better Not!

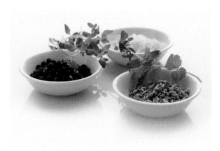

It is impossible to imagine our diet without herbs and spices. Besides the classics pepper and salt, we can find a seemingly unlimited diversity with which to refine the flavor of our meals.

Not Only Tasty but Also Good for the Body

Even though herbs, spices, and spice mixes (e.g., curry) contribute fairly little to our nutritional supply, they contain high amounts of essential oils and secondary plant substances (phytochemicals). These coloring, flavoring, and olfactory substances (e.g., flavonoids) affect the body in a variety of ways. Some stimulate the production of saliva. Others make sure that our food becomes more digestible (e.g., fennel, caraway). Or they have a positive effect on the gastrointestinal tract, liver, circulatory system, or urinary system.

You are, however, better off avoiding flavoring agents, seasonings, seasoning mixes, aromas, and flavor enhancers—or products that are made with these ingredients. In general, these contain excessive amounts of salt and additives, and the aromas are often synthetically produced. Even added so-called "natural aromas" do not live up to the expectations of many consumers. Often they are not made from the foods that they taste or smell like but from other raw materials from nature, such as wood scraps or molds.

Tip

Spices develop their greatest flavor when you heat them with the rest of the food in the pan over medium heat, but avoid overheating them because they develop a bitter taste. With herbs, it is best to add the sturdier kinds like rosemary, thyme, and bay leaves to the pot at the beginning and cook them with everything else, but without chopping them beforehand because that will release bitter-tasting compounds. More delicate herbs (basil, chervil) are best added only at the very end or sprinkled over the dish, because they lose their aroma if heated too long.

Too Much Salt Is Not Good

Salt works wonders to improve the flavor of our food but the daily allowance should not exceed 6 g (children should eat less)—the modern average lies at close to 10 g.[8] This refers to the total amount that we consume through processed products, as well as the additional salt we add to our foods in the kitchen or on the plate. People who suffer from high blood pressure and are sensitive to sodium chloride can lower their blood pressure by skimping on salt. Avoiding salt is best done by replacing it in various ways with fresh herbs and spices. We highly recommend iodized salt (except for people who are sensitive to iodine) because our natural iodine supply tends to be inadequate, which can cause iodine deficiency–related goiter.

Herbs and spices give our meals that special kick and thereby brighten our mood! For this reason, use more fresh herbs and spices, if possible organically produced and carrying one of the registered Fair Trade or small producers' labels (pp. 122 and 130).

Tip

If you do not already have an herb garden, grow your own herbs for seasoning meals or making teas on the balcony or window sill. In this way your favorite herbs are always on hand and fresh on the table.

Sweeteners from Nature

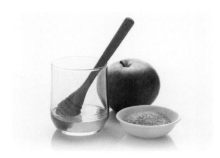

Whether in tea or coffee, in yoghurt, on bread, in cake, or as a little something sweet in between, most of us do enjoy sweet foods.

The Sensitivity Threshold for Sweetness Can Be Lowered

The sensitivity to the flavor "sweet" is more or less strongly developed in different people. We can raise, but also lower, the sensitivity threshold after which we sense sweetness. After a transitional period of several days or weeks during which we avoid sweet foods we therefore generally find that we now experience lightly sweetened foods as intensely as we previously experienced strongly sweetened ones. In turn we experience strongly sweetened products as too sweet. The strong, intrinsic flavor of sweeteners like honey or unrefined cane sugar keeps us from using too much of them. Our goal is to reduce our consumption of harmful sugars after a time of transition.

Better Avoid Isolated Sugars

Refined household sugar—whether made from cane sugar or sugar beets—belongs to the so-called isolated sugar category. This includes white and brown sugar, as well as dextrose, fructose, and so on. These contain practically no or only very few essential and beneficial nutrients. In this context brown sugar is virtually as bad as white sugar. When consumed in excess, isolated sugars promote dental caries, excess weight, and obesity. They are also linked to other disorders like type 2 diabetes, lipometabolic disorders, and arteriosclerosis. In addition, they can interfere with the digestibility of wholegrain products and cause flatulence.

Honey, Unrefined Cane Sugar, and Fruit Syrups

To cut back on sugar you can sweeten your food with fresh sweet fruit, honey, or unsulfured soaked dried fruits. Other good choices are unrefined cane sugar, unrefined beet sugar, apple syrup or other fruit syrups, agave nectar, maple syrup, or molasses—but in moderation and not in concentrated form. If these products are imported from developing countries make sure they are Fair Trade (p. 128). All the above-mentioned products are available from organic production (p. 116).

It is better to steer clear of synthetic sweeteners and products made with them, such as diet drinks and diet sweets and baked goods. Sweeteners can stimulate the appetite and induce us to consume large amounts of products sweetened with them. It should be our goal to gradually get used to a less intense sweetness in our food.

Note: More in-depth background information on the principles for a sustainable diet and a sustainable everyday life can be found in the chapter on "Sustainable Eating: The Basics" at the end of the book (from p. 111).

Tip

Rejoice in the abundant choice of fresh fruits that sweeten our lives.

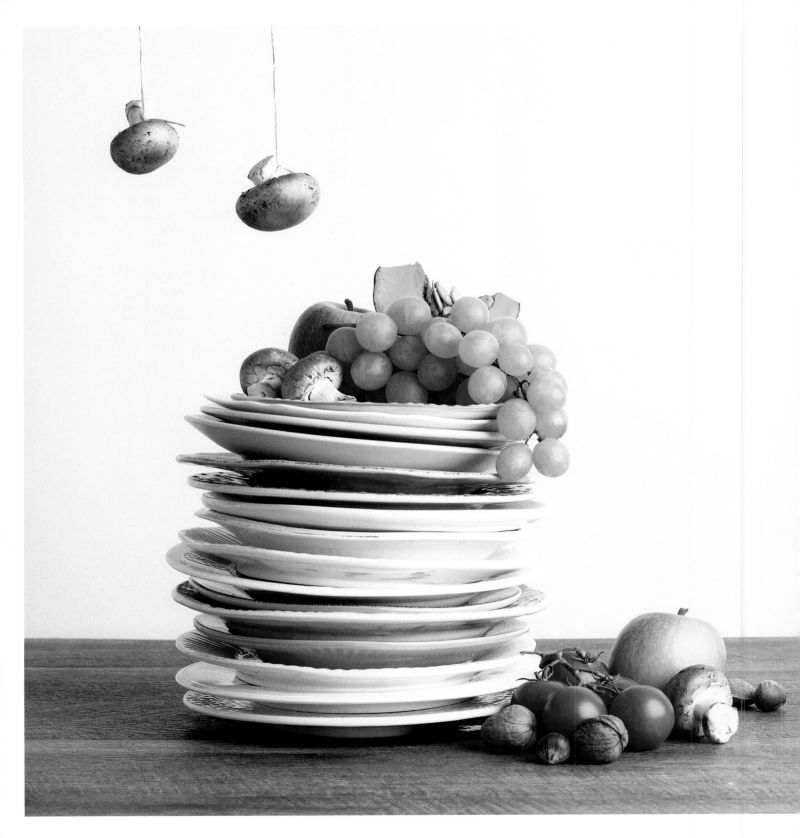

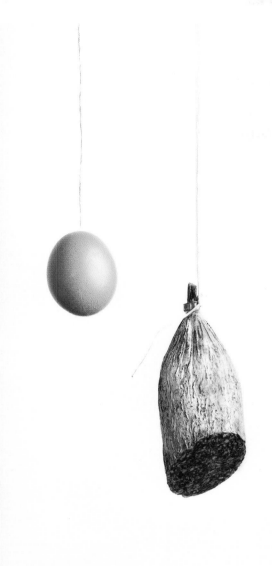

Recipes—For Cooking Sustainably

Whether it's Kohlrabi Carpaccio, Spelt Grissini with Thyme, or Chestnut Macchiato, the recipes in this chapter are diverse, with a focus on colorful vegetable-based cooking, and a handful of meat and fish dishes using, where possible, all parts of the animal.

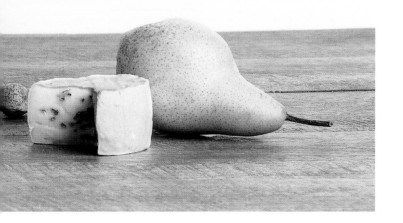

Focaccia with Tomatoes and Arugula

A focaccia made from hearty spelt, with summery toppings.

▶ For 1 baking sheet
Requires a little more time   ⊙ 50 min. + 20 min. baking time
For the dough: 20 g yeast · 200 mL warm water · salt ·
2 tbsp olive oil · 300 g wholegrain spelt flour
For the topping: 300 g tomatoes · 2 garlic cloves · 1 bunch
arugula (rocket) · 2 tbsp olive oil · salt/freshly ground pepper

– Dissolve the yeast in a little water, then add the remaining
  water with ½ tsp salt and the olive oil. Stir in the flour,
  mix well, and knead for 5 min. Let the dough rise at room
  temperature until it has roughly doubled in volume (if all
  ingredients are warm, this will take ca. 30 min.).
– Knead the dough briefly once more. Grease a round baking
  sheet or cover it with parchment paper, roll out the dough,
  place it on the sheet, and allow it to rise for another 5 min.
– Remove the stem ends of the tomatoes, score the skin
  crosswise, quickly scald them in boiling water, and peel.
  Quarter the tomatoes, remove the seeds, and cut into strips.
  Peel and crush the garlic and add to the tomatoes. Wash the
  arugula and chop it. Add to the tomatoes, and season everything with olive oil, salt, and pepper. Spread the topping
  on top of the dough.
– Let the bread rise for ca. 5 min. at room temperature. Then
  bake it at ca. 250 °C (220 °C convection oven—see conversion table p. XVIII – XIX) for 20 min.

▶ Variation
You can also wait and top the focaccia with the olive oil and
arugula after baking it. When tomatoes are not in season
you can top the focaccia with sesame, herbs, or spices instead. Just moisten the dough slightly and press the herbs
and spices in.

Nutritional value per recipe
1480 calories/ 49 g total fat/ 207 g total carbohydrates/
51 g protein

18

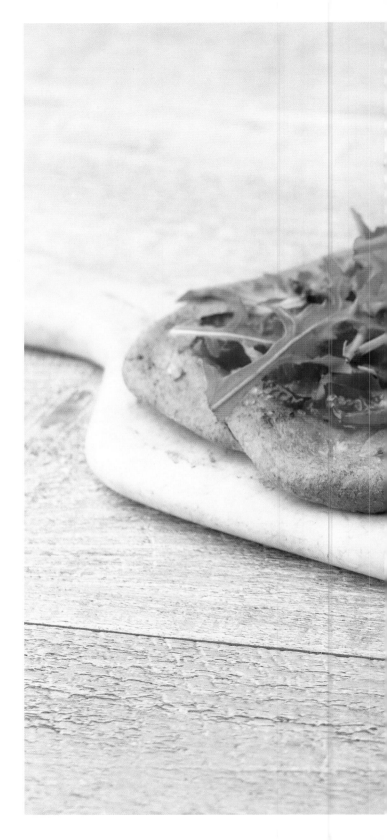

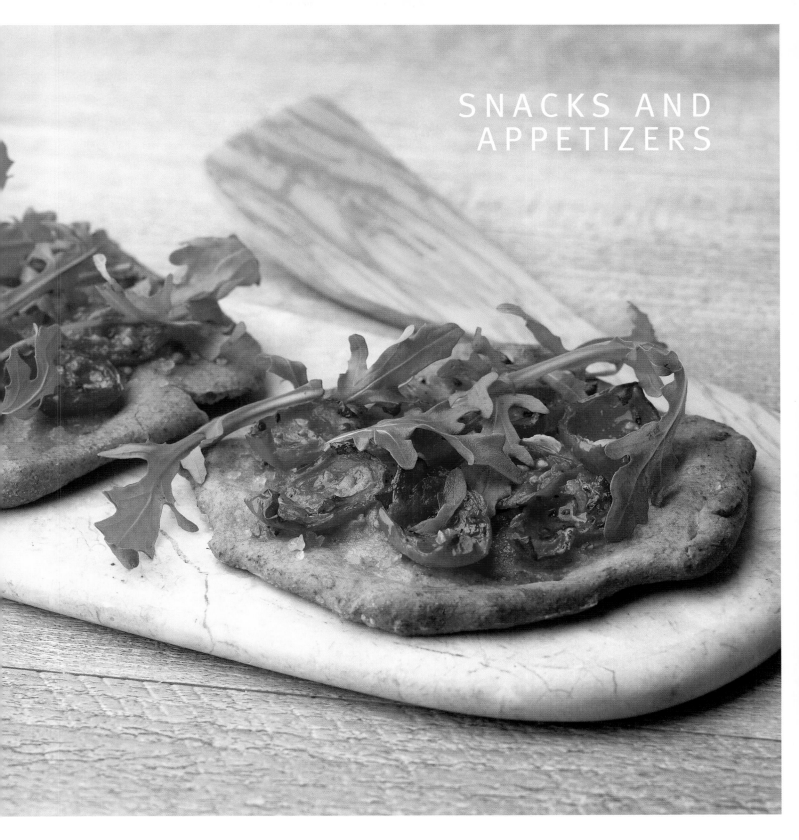

SNACKS AND APPETIZERS

Spelt Wrap with Chèvre and Lettuce
Perfect for a picnic!

► For 2 people
Good for preparing ahead of time
⏱ 30 min. + 20 min. cooking time
200 g wholegrain spelt flour · salt/freshly ground pepper ·
400 mL skim milk or vegetable broth · 1 egg · some frying oil
Ingredients for the filling: 100 g chèvre (goat cheese) · 100 g
skim quark · 1 tbsp diced chives · 2 leaves iceberg lettuce ·
½ bunch arugula · 2 tomatoes · ½ cucumber · cumin

– Mix the flour with a little salt. Stir in the milk or broth until
  you have created a smooth dough and let it rest for ca.
  30 min. Add the egg, shape into thin wraps, and fry in a pan.
– Mix the chèvre with the quark and stir the chives, salt, and
  pepper into the cheese mixture.
– Cut the lettuce and vegetables into strips and season with
  cumin, salt, and pepper. Place the cheese filling on the
  wraps, spreading it evenly. Top with the seasoned lettuce
  mixture and roll the wraps up firmly. Heat them for 10 min.
  in the oven or under the grill—they should only be lukewarm.

► Variation
Instead of the chèvre filling you can also use the Eggplant
Dip (p. 28).

► Serving suggestions
Pair the wraps with a large salad or the Black Salsify Sticks
and Ragout (p. 55). A yoghurt dip is also delicious with it.

Nutritional value per portion
640 calories/ 22 g total fat/ 81 g total carbohydrates/
29 g protein

Chèvre Baguette Au Gratin
Perfect with a large salad in the summer, or as an appetizer.

► For 4 slices
Quick to prepare   ⏱ 10 min. + 10 min. baking time
4 slices wholegrain baguette · 150 g chèvre · 60 g skim quark ·
30 g onions · 1 garlic clove · 20 g radish sprouts · cayenne

– Toast the baguette slices lightly. This can be done in the
  oven or, even easier, on the stove top. Arrange the slices on
  a metal rack and toast the bread that way.
– Purée the chèvre with the quark. Peel the onions and chop
  them finely, crush the garlic, and fold both with the radish
  sprouts into the cheese-quark mixture. Season with a little
  bit of cayenne.
– Spread the cheese mixture evenly on the toasted slices of
  bread and bake for ca. 5–10 min. in the oven.

► Variation
Also great for gratin casseroles or topping potatoes.

Nutritional values per recipe
485 calories/ 21 g total fat/ 45 g total carbohydrates/
28 g protein

FACTS
Quark
Quark is not available everywhere. In savory recipes, you
can use cottage cheese instead, but only after letting it
drain for a few minutes, otherwise it will contain too
much liquid. The resulting dish will, however, have a
slightly different consistency. Recipes that do not call for
heating the quark work well if you use firm (set) low-fat
yogurt instead. In this case, do not beat it with a mixer
(or it will turn to liquid) but stir the ingredients in with a
whisk. In Middle Eastern countries, you can replace
quark with low-fat leban or labneh.

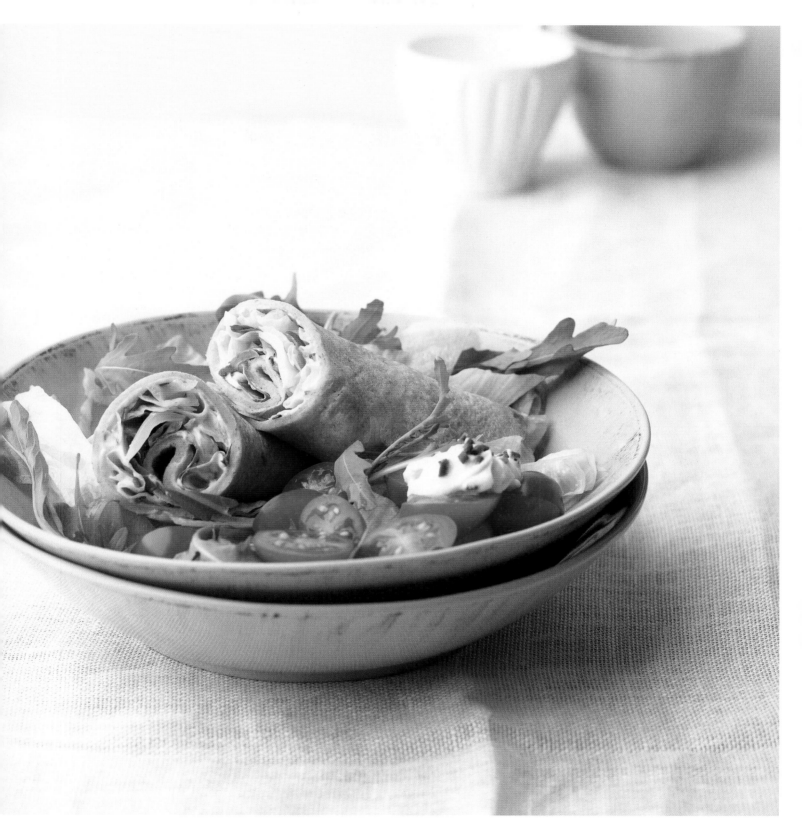

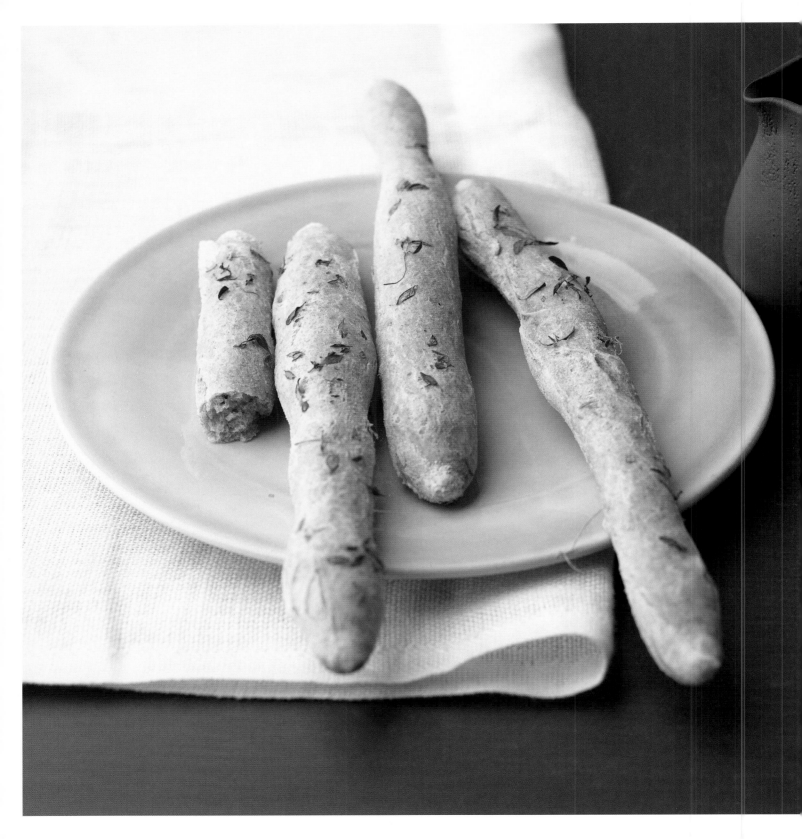

Spelt Grissini with Thyme

An Italian treat to nibble on, made from tasty spelt.

▶ For 4 people
Easy to prepare
🕐 40 min. + 10 min. baking time
20 g yeast · 200 mL water · 2 tbsp olive oil · 300 g wholegrain spelt flour · 2 twigs of thyme · salt

‒ Dissolve the yeast in a little water, then add the rest of the water with the salt and olive oil. Stir the flour into the liquid, mix well, and knead for ca. 5 min.
‒ Let the dough rise at room temperature until it has roughly doubled in volume (if all ingredients are warm, this will take ca. 30 min.).
‒ Pluck the thyme leaves off the twigs, chop the leaves, add to the dough, and briefly knead everything once more. Grease a baking sheet. Shape the grissinis like pencils and bake in a 250 °C oven (220 °C convection oven) for ca. 5–10 min. until they are crispy.

Nutritional values per recipe
1260 calories / 31 g total fat / 197 g total carbohydrates / 45 g protein

TIP
Dip the grissinis in Zucchini Crème (p. 28) or Ajvar (p. 26).

◀ Spelt Grissini with Thyme

Herb Waffles

A hearty variation, but not so high in fat.

▶ For 2–4 people
Budget-friendly
🕐 30 min. + baking time
200 g wholegrain spelt flour · 200 mL skim milk · 50 mL mineral water · 2 eggs · 1 large pinch of ground coriander · salt/freshly ground pepper · 2 tbsp fresh herbs (sage, parsley, chives)

‒ Stir the flour into the milk and water and let it rest for ca. 20 min. Separate the eggs. Add the egg yolks and spices to the flour mixture. Beat the egg whites until stiff.
‒ Wash the herbs and cut or chop them. Gently fold the stiff egg whites and herbs into the dough. Bake the dough in portions in a lightly greased waffle iron until golden brown.

▶ Serving suggestions
These waffles taste delicious, for example, with Chard Rolls (p. 29), Kohlrabi Saltimbocca (p. 57), or Zucchini Tomato Curry with Tarragon Polenta (p. 55).

Nutritional values per recipe
950 calories / 22 g total fat / 139 g total carbohydrates / 47 g protein

TIP
The waffles taste best straight from the waffle iron and can be served with many vegetable dishes.

Cheese Crackers

A savory snack, perfect with cold drinks.

▶ For 4 people
Quick to prepare
🕐 20 min. + 10 min. baking time
300 g wholewheat flour · 150 g quark · 4 tbsp olive oil · 1 egg · ½ tsp cream of tartar baking powder · pinch of salt · sage · oregano · 150 g grated Swiss cheese · 1 tsp paprika · 1 tsp caraway

‒ For the dough, stir the flour, quark, egg, baking powder, salt, oil, and sage and oregano in a bowl until well mixed and knead briefly. Roll out the dough in a thin rectangle on a floured board.
‒ Mix the cheese with the spices and sprinkle over half of the dough. Fold the other half on top, press together gently, and cut with a knife into strips that are 1 cm wide and 10 cm long.
‒ Holding the strips by both ends, twist them in opposite directions so that the cheese sticks roll up into spirals. Place them on a greased baking sheet and bake in a preheated oven at 180 °C (160 °C convection oven) for 10 min.

Nutritional values per recipe
2140 calories / 99 g total fat / 200 g total carbohydrates / 110 g protein

Muesli à la Dr. Kousmine

Great with blueberries in the summer; oranges work well in the winter.

▶ For 1 person
Budget-friendly
🕐 15 min. + 8 hours soaking time
40 g skim quark · 1 tbsp crushed grain (or flakes or sprouts) · 1 tsp flax oil · 50 g bananas · 1 – 4 tbsp orange juice (optional) · 80 g apple · 30 g seasonal fruit · 1 tsp oilseeds, soaked and crushed

– Crush the grains and soak them in 3 tsp water overnight. Purée the quark with the oil, bananas, and some of the juice. Grate the apples and add to the quark mixture together with the seasonal fruit, grains, and oilseeds.

▶ Variation
You can vary this recipe with different types of fruit—depending on the season—or grains and spices. If you use oats always use them fresh and grind finely or crush into flakes but do not soak them, otherwise they turn bitter. Spelt and other grains can either be finely ground and added directly to the muesli, or crushed and soaked in water overnight or sprouted.

Nutritional values per portion
250 calories/ 8 g total fat/ 34 g total carbohydrates/ 9 g protein

Muesli with Peach Crème

A wonderful summer muesli—best with ripe peaches.

▶ For 2 people
Easy to prepare
🕐 15 min. + 8 hours soaking time
2 tbsp spelt · 1 tbsp sunflower seeds 2 peaches · 1 tbsp white almond paste · 2 apples

– The day before, coarsely crush the spelt and soak overnight in 50 mL water. Dry-roast the sunflower seeds in a pan until they become fragrant.
– Cut the peaches in half, remove the pits, dice, and purée with the almond paste. Grate the apples and add. Lastly, mix in the roasted sunflower seeds and the crushed spelt.

▶ Variation
Even in other seasons you can always find suitable kinds of seasonal fruit.

Nutritional values per portion
270 calories/ 9 g total fat/ 40 g total carbohydrates/ 6 g protein

Herb Muesli

This muesli is also delicious as a sandwich spread and even tastes good with boiled or baked potatoes.

▶ For 2 people
Quick to prepare
🕐 10 min.
100 g skim quark · 2 tbsp olive oil · 1 tomato · 1 miniature cucumber (ca. 100 g) · 2 sprigs of basil · 2 tbsp sprouted grain · salt/freshly ground pepper

– Stir the skim quark with the olive oil until smooth. Dice the tomato and cucumber into small cubes. Pluck the basil leaves and chop finely then mix them with the sprouted grain into the other ingredients. Season everything with salt and pepper.

Nutritional values per recipe
150 calories/ 10 g total fat/ 5 g total carbohydrates/ 8 g protein

Chocolate Spread

Kids love to help with the preparation of this dish!

▶ For 1 jar
Easy to prepare   ⊙ 10 min. + 3 min. cooking time
250 mL milk · 3 tbsp cocoa powder · pinch of natural vanilla ·
pinch of salt · 30 g polenta · 50 g finely ground hazelnuts ·
1 tbsp almond oil · 60 g honey

▬ Bring the milk to a boil with the cocoa powder, vanilla, and
salt. Stir in the polenta and ground hazelnuts and cook for
2–3 min. until you get a porridge-like consistency.
▬ Stir the oil and honey into the hot mixture, adjust the seasonings, and purée finely with a blender. Pour into a glass
jar and let it cool off.

▶ Variation
You can use hazelnut oil instead of almond oil but the
chocolate spread tastes even more delicious with the
almond oil. The reason for this is that it contains a lot of
polyunsaturated fatty acids—similar to hazelnut and walnut oil—but tastes slightly sweet. It is therefore an ideal
choice for sweet dishes. Make sure that you buy sweet
almond oil, and not bitter almond oil.

Nutritional values per recipe
830 calories/ 46 g total fat/ 73 g total carbohydrates/
32 g protein

Strawberry Spread

All the valuable ingredients in the fruits are preserved.

▶ For 1 jar
Easy to prepare   ⊙ 10 min. + 1 hour sitting time
50 g dried apple rings · 200 g strawberries · honey,
as needed

▬ Coarsely chop the apple rings and strawberries. Combine
and let the fruit sit for 1 hour to soften the apple rings a
little. Then purée everything and sweeten with a little
honey, depending on the sweetness of the berries. If the
spread is not perfectly smooth at this point, wait a while
and then purée it a second time.

▶ Other combinations
▬ Sour cherries and dried figs
▬ Fresh plums and dried plums, with a little cinnamon

Nutritional values per recipe
190 calories/ 2 g total fat/ 39 g total carbohydrates/
2 g protein

Any ripe fruits can be used for this kind of fruit spread.
The amount of dried fruit depends on the water content
of the fresh fruit. This fruit spread can be stored in the
fridge for 1 week.

FACTS

Vanilla

Many of the recipes use natural vanilla in powdered form. To prepare this ingredient freeze a whole vanilla bean and then grind
it finely or purée it. This method has the advantage that you are using the entire bean and that you can also use it for dishes
that are not cooked. In the standard method, you cook the entire vanilla bean and then scrape out the inside. In uncooked
dishes, however, this means that you can only scrape out the pulp and then place the remaining pod in honey, unrefined
sugar, or fruit juice concentrate to flavor these sweeteners with the empty pod, in order to use the entire vanilla bean.
Vanilla sugar or powder is made with artificial vanillin and therefore not desirable.

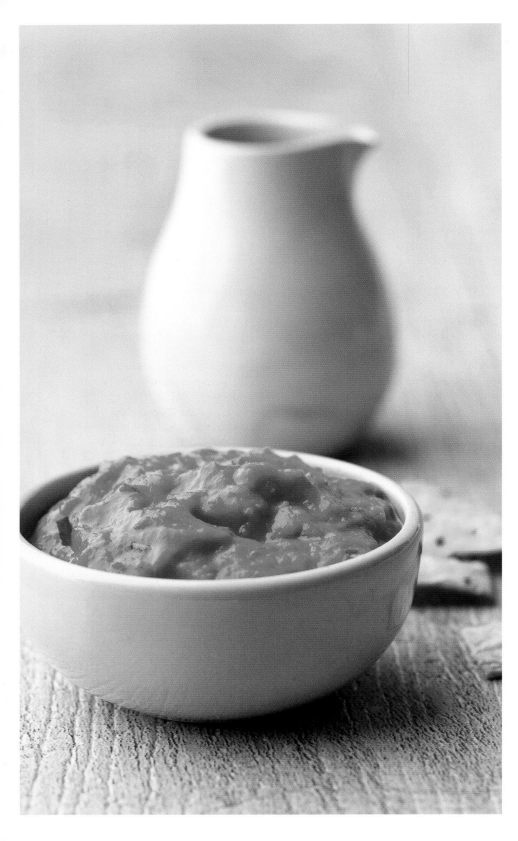

Ajvar

Ajvar is a flavorful red pepper crème, originally from the Balkans.

▶ **For 4 people**
Requires a little more time
⊙ **20 min. + 25 min. roasting time**
200 g red bell peppers · **150 g** eggplants (aubergines) · **100 g** tomatoes · **100 g** onions · **1 tbsp** olive oil · **1 garlic clove** · a little fresh chili powder · salt

- Roast the peppers and eggplants in a 180 °C oven (160 °C convection oven) for ca. 25 min, then peel them. Remove the stem end of the tomatoes, score the skin, and steam for 1 min. or poach briefly in boiling water. Rinse quickly under cold water, peel and quarter.
- Peel the onions, dice and sauté briefly in olive oil. Then add the quartered tomatoes, crushed garlic, and chili and sauté again briefly. Purée everything together in a blender and season with salt.

▶ **Serving suggestions**
Ajvar works well as a spread or savory condiment for all sorts of things. It keeps for 7 days in the refrigerator.

Nutritional values per recipe
200 calories/ 11 g total fat/ 17 g total carbohydrates/ 6 g protein

TIP
To save time, you can roast all the vegetables in the oven and then purée them with the other ingredients.

Lentil Spread

A light vegetarian spread low in fat.

▶ For 4 people
Good for preparing ahead of time
🕙 15 min. + 20 min. cooking time
50 g onions · 125 g carrots · 1 twig of marjoram · 1 tsp olive oil · 125 g red lentils · 500 mL vegetable broth · 1 tbsp tomato paste · 2 tbsp raspberry vinegar · 2 tbsp almond oil · salt/freshly ground pepper

– Peel the onions and carrots, chop and sauté them briefly with the marjoram in the olive oil. Add the red lentils, stir in the tomato paste, and deglaze with the vegetable broth and raspberry vinegar.
– Cook everything until all ingredients are soft and the liquid has evaporated. Pour into a blender, add the almond oil, season with salt and pepper, and purée.

Nutritional values per recipe
670 calories/ 27 g total fat/ 73 g total carbohydrates/ 31 g protein

Tip

You can make this spread richer by adding 150 g quark or sour cream. It keeps in the fridge for 4–5 days.

Squash and Chèvre Spread

With a full savory flavor and not too heavy.

▶ For 4 people
Easy to prepare
🕙 10 min. + 20 min. cooking time
1 small onion · ½ tsp olive oil · 500 g Hokkaido squash (i.e., red kuri) · 1 tbsp cider vinegar · 1 large pinch cumin · salt/freshly ground pepper · 1 tbsp mustard · 100 g chèvre (or any other fresh cheese)

– Peel and finely dice the onion. Sauté over medium heat in the olive oil. Wash the squash, remove the seeds, and cut into 0.5-cm cubes without removing the peel. Add to the onion and sauté until the squash is very soft.
– Season everything with the cider vinegar, cumin, salt, and pepper. Stir in the mustard and fresh chèvre and season again to taste. Put in a suitable container and keep in the refrigerator.

Nutritional values per recipe
330 calories/ 15 g total fat/ 29 g total carbohydrates/ 18 g protein

Tip

This spread tastes deliciously fresh if you use yoghurt instead of the chèvre. In addition, you can also purée the spread until completely smooth.

Puréed Beans

A hearty accompaniment for vegetable dishes.

▶ For 2 people
Budget-friendly
🕙 1 hour + 8 hours soaking time
100 g dry white beans · bay leaf · thyme · 50 g potatoes · 2 tbsp milk · truffle oil, salt/freshly ground pepper cumin

– Soak the beans overnight in cold water. Cook the beans with the bay leaf and thyme until soft. Alternatively, you can use 300 g cooked beans. Steam the potatoes in the skin, then peel and mash them with a fork. Purée the soft beans, add to the mashed potatoes, and beat with the milk and a few drops of truffle oil. Season with the spices.

▶ Serving suggestions
A delicious accompaniment for vegetable dishes like Eggplant Piccata (p. 61), but also good simply with steamed vegetables.

Nutritional values per portion
190 calories/ 2 g total fat/ 28 g total carbohydrates/ 15 g protein

SNACKS AND APPETIZERS

Eggplant Dip

This dip goes particularly well with freshly baked flatbread.

▶ For 4 people
Easy to prepare
⏱ 15 min. + 30 min. cooking time
100 g quark · 250 g eggplant · 2 garlic cloves · 50 g cream cheese · 2 tbsp lemon juice · salt/freshly ground pepper

– Drain the quark in a strainer. Pierce the eggplant with a knife all over and roast with the peeled garlic cloves in a 160 °C oven (150 °C convection oven) for ca. 30 min. Then cut the eggplant in half and scoop out the flesh with a spoon.
– Chop the eggplant coarsely and purée with the other ingredients in a blender or with a stick blender to create a spreadable crème. Season to taste.

Nutritional values per recipe
295 calories/ 17 g total fat/ 13 g total carbohydrates/ 23 g protein

Zucchini Crème

Wonderful with very young zucchinis that don't have hard seeds.

▶ For 4 people
Budget-friendly
⏱ 10 min. + 15 min. cooking time
100 g potatoes · 2 zucchinis · 1 onion 1 garlic clove · 1 tsp olive oil · 1 rosemary twig · salt/freshly ground pepper · 50 g skim quark or sour cream · juice from ½ lemon

– Steam the potatoes in the skin and then peel them. Cube the zucchinis. Chop the onions finely, crush the garlic clove. Sauté the garlic, zucchinis, rosemary, and onion in the olive oil over medium heat until the zucchini pieces are soft.
– Mash the potatoes, add to the zucchinis, and season with salt and pepper. Take out the rosemary and purée everything else. Stir in the quark and season with the lemon juice and spices.

Nutritional values per recipe
255 calories/ 6 g total fat/ 30 g total carbohydrates/ 16 g protein

TIP
It is quicker if you use boiled potatoes from the day before. The zucchini crème keeps for 4–5 days in the fridge.

Chickpea Snack

A low-fat snack—perfect for nibbling.

▶ For 2 people
Easy to prepare
⏱ 50 min. + 8 hours soaking time
100 g chickpeas · 400 mL water · 2 bay leaves · 2 cloves · 5 peppercorns and 5 juniper berries · tamari · paprika

– Soak the chickpeas overnight in the water. Before cooking them add the bay leaves, cloves, peppercorns, and juniper berries. Cook the chickpeas until soft.
– Put the cooked chickpeas on a baking sheet and roast in a preheated oven for ca. 20 min. at 220 °C (200 °C convection oven). Season the crunchy chickpeas with tamari and paprika and serve immediately—still warm.

▶ Variation
You can create a tasty variation by seasoning with wasabi (Japanese horseradish) and honey.

Nutritional values per recipe
320 calories/ 6 g total fat/ 45 g total carbohydrates/ 20 g protein

TIP
You can also cook the chickpeas a day in advance. It is easiest to add the spices to the chickpeas in a disposable tea strainer. That way it is not as much trouble to remove the spices later.

Chard Rolls

Very Italian, with pine nuts and raisins.

▶ For 2 people
Easy to prepare 🕙 20 min. + 20 min. cooking time
8 whole chard leaves · 1 onion · 20 g pine nuts · 20 g raisins ·
1 tbsp olive oil · 1 tbsp raspberry vinegar · salt/freshly
ground pepper · nutmeg · coriander · 1 tbsp tomato paste

- Cut out the stems of the chard and blanch the 4 prettiest
  leaves. Cut the chard stems and onions into strips and
  sauté in a little oil. Cut the remaining leaves into strips and
  add to the stems shortly before these are completely soft.
- Roast the pine nuts in an ungreased pan and add to the
  chard, along with the raisins. Season everything with the
  spices and vinegar and thicken it with the tomato paste.
- Flatten out the blanched leaves and season them with a
  little salt and pepper. Spread the filling on the leaves, fold
  the ends over, and roll them up. Place the chard rolls in an
  ovenproof dish and heat for 10 min. in the oven before
  serving.

▶ Serving suggestions
The rolls taste delicious with wholegrain pancakes or
waffles. Also great with eggplant or yoghurt dip.

Nutritional values per portion
170 calories/ 11 g total fat/ 11 g total carbohydrates/
6 g protein

Tip

Alternatively, you can heat the chard rolls in a pan
with a little liquid or by steaming them.

Lentil Croquettes

These croquettes are high in protein and complex
carbohydrates.

▶ For 2 people
Budget-friendly 🕙 15 min. + 45 min. cooking time
100 g lentils · 200 mL water · 2 bay leaves · 50 g carrots ·
50 g celeriac · 50 g leek · tamari · cumin · pepper · 3 tbsp
wholegrain breadcrumbs · 1 egg · 2 tbsp wholewheat flour

- Put the lentils in a pot with the bay leaves and boil in the
  water until soft. When done, all the water should have
  evaporated.
- Finely grate the carrots and celeriac and finely chop the
  leek. Brown the vegetables in a pan and season with cumin, pepper, and tamari. Add everything to the soft lentils
  and let them sit for 5 min. Using 2 spoons or the palm of
  your hand, shape the mixture into small dumplings and
  put them on a plate.
- Mix the egg with the flour. When the dumplings have
  cooled off a little, roll them first in the egg-flour mixture
  and then in the breadcrumbs. Fry them in a pan over medium heat or bake them in the oven.

▶ Serving suggestions
Quite delicious with a squash stir-fry.

Nutritional values per portion
280 calories/ 4 g total fat/ 41 g total carbohydrates/
19 g protein

FACTS

Tamari

Tamari is a fermented seasoning sauce made from soy
beans and sea salt–slightly stronger in smell and taste
than ordinary soy sauce.

Asparagus Mousse

Most likely you have never eaten asparagus as a mousse before!

▶ For 2 people
Requires a little more time
🕐 30 min. + 40 min. cooking time
150 g potatoes · 1 kg white asparagus · 50 g skim quark · 1 tbsp almond oil · 2 eggs · salt · cayenne

— Steam the potatoes in the skin and peel them. Peel the asparagus. Cut the asparagus tips off at about 3 cm and set them aside. Steam the rest of the asparagus until soft. Purée the cooked asparagus, potatoes, quark, eggs, half the oil, and a pinch each of salt and pepper, then adjust the seasonings again.
— Use the remaining oil to grease an ovenproof dish and pour the mousse into it. Cook over steam or in the oven with water in an ovenproof dish for ca. 25 min. Right before serving, sauté the asparagus tips in a little olive oil and season with salt and a hint of cayenne. Let the mousse cool a little and invert onto a plate. Serve with the asparagus tips.

▶ Serving suggestions

Tastes great with potatoes or red potato pearls: to prepare these, boil 300 g potato balls (made by scooping out raw potatoes with a melon baller) in 400 mL beet juice until soft. Serve everything together with Base Sauce (see p. 48), seasoned with a little almond oil and tarragon.

Nutritional values per portion
290 calories/ 11 g total fat/ 23 g total carbohydrates/ 22 g protein

TIP

Use boiled potatoes from the day before.

Leek Mousse with Apple Vinaigrette

A nice appetizer or a light dinner in winter.

▶ For 2 people
Budget-friendly
🕐 40 min. + 2 hours cooling time
300 g leek (white parts) · 150 mL water · 1 tsp agar-agar · salt/freshly ground pepper · 125 g cream cheese · cayenne · 2 tbsp canola oil · 1 tbsp white wine vinegar or lemon juice · 50 g apple · freshly grated horseradish

— Clean and wash the leek, cut into strips, and sauté lightly. Cook with the water, agar-agar, and a little salt in a covered pot for about 20 min. until soft. Then refrigerate everything for at least 2 hours. Finely purée the solid leek mixture in a blender and fold in the fresh cheese.
— Mix the canola oil with the vinegar. Chop the apple very finely, add to the dressing, grate some horseradish into it, and season with salt and pepper. To serve, scoop out the mousse in the shape of little dumplings or fill small glasses and drizzle with the apple vinaigrette. You can also garnish this dish with small cubes of cooked beets.

Nutritional values per portion
365 calories/ 30 g total fat/ 11 g total carbohydrates/ 12 g protein

TIP

If you are unable to chop the apple so finely, grate it whole or purée it with the oil and vinegar.

▶ Leek mousse with apple vinaigrette

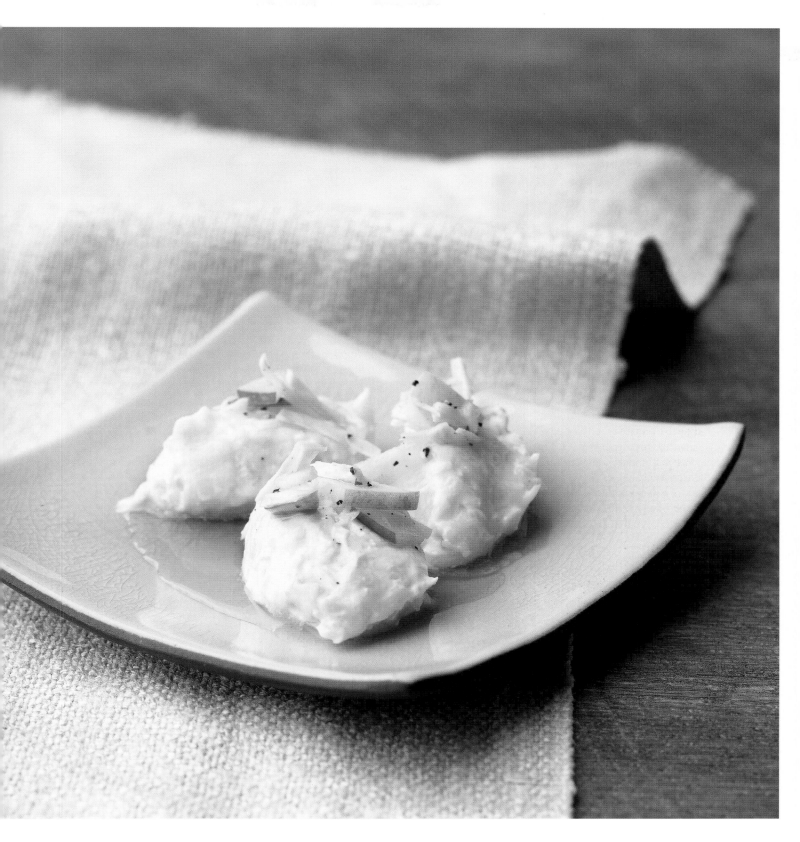

Beet Mousse

An elegant appetizer or great side dish for smoked fish.

▶ For 2 people
Good for preparing ahead of time
🕐 15 min. + 1 hour cooking time
300 g beets · freshly grated horse-radish · 50 g quark · 1 tbsp white balsamic or white wine vinegar · ground caraway seed · salt/freshly ground pepper

— Cook the beets for ca. 25 min. until soft. The beets are done when you can easily insert a knife and pull it back out without resistance. Let the beets cool down briefly and peel them.
— Now cut them into small pieces, place in a blender, add a little grated horseradish, and blend with the quark and spices. Season with bal-samic vinegar and, if needed, adjust the seasonings.

Nutritional values per portion
80 calories/ 0 g total fat/ 13 g total carbohydrates/ 6 g protein

TIP

For a special occasion it is a nice idea to serve a trio of beets, consisting of this mousse, the Kohlrabi Carpaccio (p. 40), and the Beet Macchiato (p. 46).

Jerusalem Artichoke Mousse

A Jerusalem artichoke mousse and beet mousse duo looks beautiful.

▶ For 2 people
Easy to prepare
🕐 10 min. + 20 min. cooking time
300 g Jerusalem artichokes · 50 g leek (white parts) · 1 tsp olive oil · 1 tbsp walnut oil · salt/freshly ground pepper · lemon juice

— Wash and finely chop the Jerusalem artichoke tubers and the leek. Heat the olive oil lightly in a pan, add the vegetables and a little water, and cook with a closed lid until soft.
— When done the entire liquid should have evaporated. Put the vegetables in a blender, add the walnut oil, salt, pepper, and a little lemon juice, and purée everything until very smooth. Season generously.

Nutritional values per portion
120 calories/ 8 g total fat/ 7 g total carbohydrates/ 4 g protein

TIP

Jerusalem artichoke tubers do not need to be peeled.

Zucchini Turrets

Taste best when made with young zucchinis.

▶ For 2 people
Easy to prepare
🕐 20 min. + 30 min. sitting time
1 tomato · 1 tsp honey · 50 g cashew nuts · 1 tbsp chopped basil · salt/freshly ground pepper · garlic · 200 g zucchinis

— Wash the tomato, remove the stem end, and purée with the honey. Finely grind the cashew nuts, add the tomato, and blend until smooth. Season everything with the basil, garlic, and the spices.
— Slice the zucchinis evenly, spread the tomato-cashew mixture on the slices and stack them on top of each other. Allow the turrets to sit to ab-sorb the flavors for about half an hour.

Nutritional values per portion
215 calories/ 12 g total fat/ 18 g total carbohydrates/ 8 g protein

Italian Antipasti
Delicious cold or warm!

▶ For 2 people
Good for preparing ahead of time
⏱ 10 min. + 20 min. baking time
1 zucchini · 1 red bell pepper · 1 yellow bell pepper · 1 onion
salt/freshly ground pepper · juice and peel from 1 lemon ·
2 rosemary twigs · thyme · 3 tbsp balsamic vinegar · 2 tbsp
olive oil

— Cut the zucchinis into 1-cm-wide slices. Slice the bell peppers in half, remove the seeds, and cut into 1-cm-wide
  strips. Cut the onion in half and slice into even sections no
  wider than 1 cm at their thickest spot.
— Arrange the prepared vegetables on a baking sheet and
  season with salt and pepper. Sprinkle the lemon juice and
  peel, thyme, and rosemary on the vegetables.
— Bake the vegetables for ca. 20 min. in a 170 °C oven
  (150 °C convection oven). Then remove the herbs, pour the
  vinegar and oil onto the vegetables while they are still hot,
  mix, and arrange on a platter.

Nutritional values per portion
160 calories/ 11 g total fat/ 12 g total carbohydrates/
4 g protein

Tip

**Drizzle the oil and vinegar on the vegetables when these
are still hot so that the flavors can soak in better. You can
keep the antipasti in the fridge for several days.**

Asparagus Confection
A beautiful treat for guests!

▶ For 2 people
Easy to prepare
⏱ 45 min. + 15 min. cooking time
100 g skim quark · 100 g cream cheese · 300 g white asparagus · 1 tsp tarragon · salt/freshly ground pepper · 20 g pine
nuts · 3 slices of crispbread · lemon basil

— Drain the quark in a strainer for 30 min. and whip with the
  cream cheese. Peel the asparagus and use a grater to grate
  into fine slivers. Leave the tips ca. 5 cm long and steam
  these until soft. Pluck the tarragon leaves, mince, and fold
  with the grated asparagus, salt, and pepper into the quark
  mixture.
— Briefly roast the pine nuts, let them cool, and grind with
  the crispbread in a nut grinder or cheese grater. Pluck the
  lemon basil, mince, and mix with the pine nuts and crispbread. Put this mixture in a deep dish.
— Shape the quark-asparagus mixture into balls or scoop out
  dumplings with 2 spoons, roll these in the breadcrumb
  coating, and arrange on a platter. Serve with the steamed
  asparagus tips.

▶ Variation
If you don't like raw asparagus you can steam it briefly,
but it has to be very much al dente otherwise you won't
be able to grate it.

Nutritional values per recipe
675 calories/ 43 g total fat/ 33 g total carbohydrates/
39 g protein

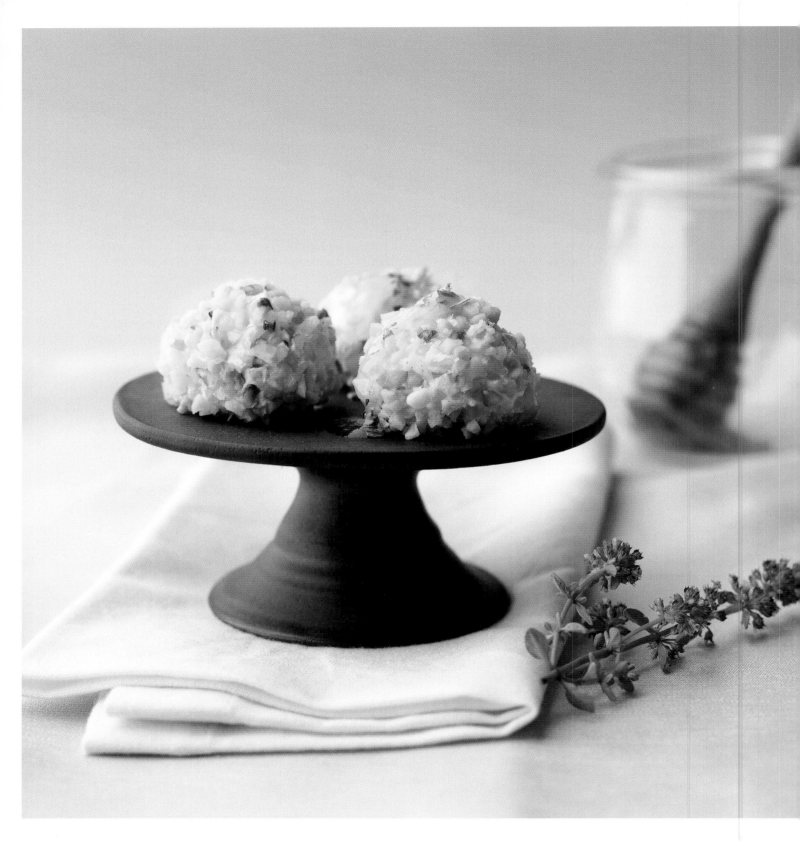

Chèvre Balls with Thyme Honey

These little balls are a nice-looking appetizer.

▶ For 2 –4 people
Quick to prepare 🕐 20 min. + 2 hours steeping time
2 twigs of thyme · 100 g wild honey · 100 g skim quark ·
200 g chèvre · salt/freshly ground pepper · 20 g walnuts

▬ To make the thyme honey, pluck the thyme leaves, chop
finely, and mix into the honey. The honey should steep for
at least 2 hours, but can also steep like this for several days.
▬ For the balls, place the quark in a strainer and let it drain,
then mix with the chèvre and season with salt and pepper.
Grate or chop the walnuts very finely.
▬ Form small balls of about 15 g each and roll in the ground
nuts. Before serving, drizzle them with the thyme honey
or dip them halfway in.

Nutritional values per recipe
855 calories/ 40 g total fat/ 88 g total carbohydrates/
34 g protein

FACTS

Ingenious Combinations with Red Cabbage Sorbet

You can achieve the best flavor by marinating the red
cabbage and apple overnight. Incidentally, the Red
Cabbage Sorbet is nothing but your standard recipe for
cooking red cabbage. You just add the almond oil at the
end. Thus you can simply cook normal red cabbage and
freeze part of it after mixing it with the appropriate
amount of oil. The sorbet gives many hearty dishes a
great kick, for example, the Chestnut Soufflé (p. 50)
or the Celeriac Cordon Bleu (p. 69), but you can also
serve it with meat dishes.

Red Cabbage Sorbet

This sorbet provides just the right kick for all sorts of hearty
dishes.

▶ For 2 people
Good for preparing ahead of time
🕐 1 hour + 2 –4 hours freezing time
500 g fresh red cabbage · 1 apple · 50 mL apple juice · clove ·
cinnamon · bay leaf · 1 onion · 50 g potatoes · salt/freshly
ground pepper · 2 tbsp almond oil

▬ Rinse the red cabbage, clean and cut into strips. Cut the
apple into quarters, core and thinly slice it. Marinate in the
apple juice and herbs and spices. Sauté the onions briefly,
add the cabbage, and cook until soft. Peel the potatoes and
grate very finely into the cabbage. Cook for another
10 min.—this thickens the cabbage—and season again with
salt and pepper.
▬ You can adjust the consistency with a little vegetable broth
or apple juice. Mix in the almond oil and pour everything
into a mold, let it cool, and freeze it. Crush the frozen cabbage in a food processor or in a meat grinder. Fluff it up
with a whisk and place on the plate immediately before
serving.

▶ Info
Compared with other oils, almond oil does not have a very
strong flavor and is slightly sweet, which works well for
this recipe.

Nutritional values per portion
225 calories/ 11 g total fat/ 27 g total carbohydrates/
5 g protein

Du Puy Lentils with Radicchio

This salad tastes even better if you wait a few hours before eating.

▶ For 2–4 people
Requires a little more time
⊙ 15 min. + 45 min. cooking time
200 g du Puy lentils (or brown lentils) · **1** rosemary twig · **2** garlic cloves · **3 tbsp** olive oil · **1 tsp** mustard · **4 tbsp** balsamic vinegar · salt/freshly ground pepper · cayenne · **100 g** radicchio · **30 g** arugula

- Cook the lentils with the rosemary and garlic in 500 mL unsalted water until soft—this takes about 30–45 min. Prepare a marinade with the balsamic vinegar, olive oil, mustard, and spices, and stir this into the cooked lentils.
- Cut the radicchio and arugula into fine strips and fold under the cooled lentils. Adjust the seasoning again.

Nutritional values per portion
450 calories/ 17 g total fat/ 48 g total carbohydrates/ 25 g protein

TIP

The salad is a little much for 2 people but stores well, for example, to take with you to the office.

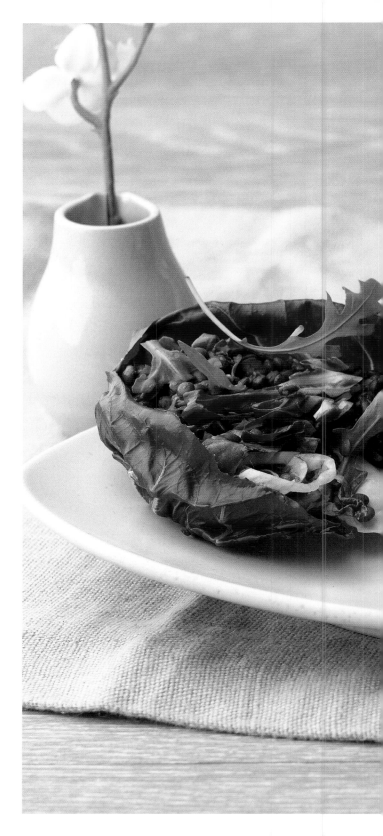

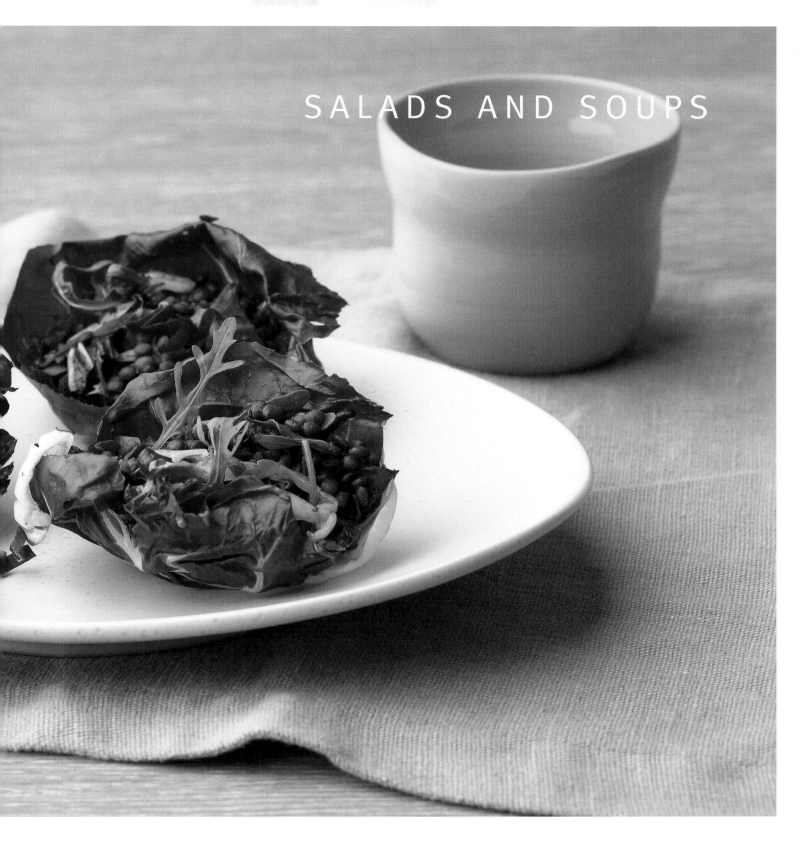

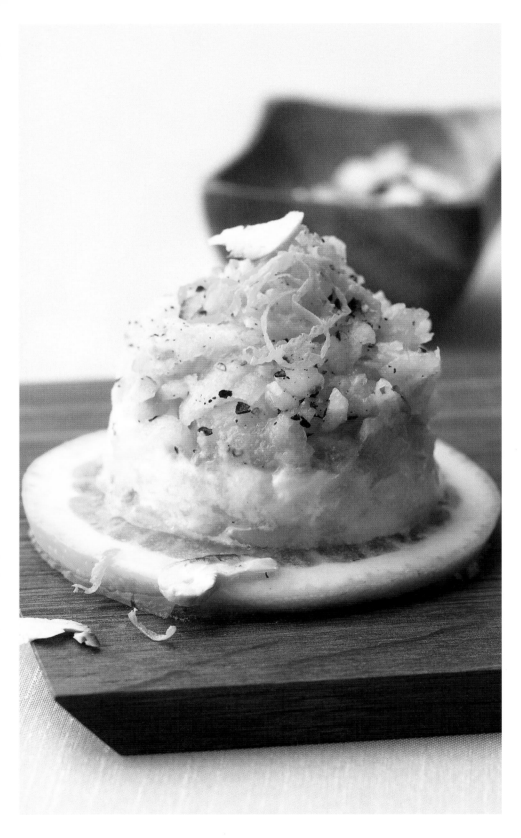

Broccoli, Pear, and Cashew Salad

Fruity and nutty—a fine raw food treat.

▶ For 2 people
Easy to prepare
⏱ 15 min.

30 g cashew nuts · 1 tbsp hazelnut oil ·
1 tbsp raspberry vinegar · juice from half
an orange · salt/freshly ground pepper ·
50 g low-fat yoghurt · 250 g broccoli ·
100 g pear

— Roast the cashews in an ungreased pan
and chop finely. Stir all the remaining
ingredients together except for the
broccoli and pear, and add the cashew
nuts to this.
— Use a knife to peel the broccoli stems.
Using a grater, grate the broccoli directly into the marinade. Core the pear
and grate it into the marinade. Mix
everything and, if necessary, adjust the
seasonings.

Nutritional values per portion
230 calories/ 13 g total fat/ 16 g total
carbohydrates/ 9 g protein

Endive Orange Salad

A typical winter salad, also delicious with blood oranges.

► For 2 people
Budget-friendly ⊘ 10 min.
1 orange · 50 g yoghurt · 50 g butter-milk · freshly grated horseradish · honey · tomato paste · salt · 200 g endive

– Cut the orange in half. Squeeze one half and peel the other. Prepare the marinade by combining the yoghurt, buttermilk, a little horse-radish, orange juice, a little honey, tomato paste, and the salt.
– Cut the endive in half, remove the core, and cut into thin strips. Cut the remaining orange half likewise into thin strips and add together with the endive to the marinade.

Nutritional values per portion
75 calories/ 1 g total fat/ 11 g total carbohydrates/ 4 g protein

Fresh Asparagus Salad

You can also serve the avocado sauce with cooked asparagus.

► For 2 people
Requires a little more time
⊘ 20 min. + 10 min. cooking time
500 g white asparagus · 50 g avoca-do · 2 tbsp almond oil · 2 tbsp lemon juice · 4 tbsp asparagus stock · salt/ freshly ground pepper · 100 g pea pods (young peas in the pod) · 100 g radishes · 1 tbsp dill

– Peel the asparagus. Cut off the tips at ca. 3 cm and boil in water with a little lemon juice and salt until soft. Purée the avocado, almond oil, lemon juice, and asparagus stock. Season with salt and pepper.
– Grate the raw asparagus stalks with a vegetable slicer into fine slices and cut the pea pods into fine strips and the radishes into fine slivers. Add everything immediately to the sauce and season to taste. Pluck the dill, chop finely, and add as well. Garnish the salad with the cooked asparagus tips.

Nutritional values per portion
210 calories/ 14 g total fat/ 13 g total carbohydrates/ 8 g protein

Celeriac Salad with Nut Dressing

A hearty winter salad, substantial and yet refined with hazelnuts.

► For 2 people
Budget-friendly ⊘ 10 min.
1 orange · 50 g hazelnuts (or mixed nuts) · 2 tbsp salad oil (a combina-tion of primarily canola oil, sesame oil, pumpkin seed oil, and a little olive oil) · 2 tbsp white wine vinegar · salt/freshly ground pepper · 300 g blemish-free celeriac root

– Cut the orange in half. Squeeze one half, peel the other half, and cut into small pieces. Lightly toast the ha-zelnuts and grind or chop finely. For the marinade, stir the remain-ing ingredients together.
– Peel the celeriac root, grate it very finely directly into the marinade, mix it in, let everything soak for a little while, and season to taste.

Nutritional values per portion
300 calories/ 26 g total fat/ 8 g total carbohydrates/ 7 g protein

TIP
Because of the canola oil, the mixture contains a lot of omega-3 fatty acids, while the other oils round out the flavor.

Kohlrabi Apple Salad

With high-quality basic ingredients, salads can be simple but delicious.

▶ **For 2 people**
Quick to prepare ⏱ 10 min.
3 tbsp white balsamic vinegar ·
4 tbsp canola oil · salt/freshly ground pepper · 200 g kohlrabi · 100 g apple

— Put the vinegar, oil, salt, and pepper in a bowl and stir. Peel the kohlrabi and grate it directly into the salad dressing, mixing it in. Also grate the apple without removing the peel, mix it in, and season to taste.

▶ **Variation**
The dressing also tastes great with mustard and herbs.

Nutritional values per portion
235 calories / 20 g total fat / 11 g total carbohydrates / 2 g protein

Kohlrabi Carpaccio

Tastes wonderful with shaved Parmesan or pecorino.

▶ **For 2 people**
Requires a little more time
⏱ 15 min. + 1 hour soaking time
4 tbsp pumpkin seed oil · 2 tbsp white wine vinegar · salt/freshly ground pepper · 200 g kohlrabi · 1 tbsp pumpkin seeds · ½ bunch chives

— Combine the pumpkin seed oil, vinegar, salt, and pepper. Peel the kohlrabi and shave into very thin slivers. Arrange these slices fan-like on a platter, brush with the marinade, and let everything soak for at least 1 hour.
— Toast the pumpkin seeds, cut the chives into small rolls, and sprinkle both on the kohlrabi before serving.

Nutritional values per portion
235 calories / 23 g total fat / 4 g total carbohydrates / 4 g protein

TIP
You will get the thinnest slices with a truffle slicer.

Beet Salad

Beets are also tasty raw!

▶ **For 2 people**
Quick to prepare ⏱ 10 min.
2 tbsp walnut oil · 50 mL apple juice · 2 tbsp cider vinegar · salt/freshly ground pepper · caraway · a small amount of fresh horseradish · 300 g beets · 1 apple

— Prepare the marinade by combining the oil, apple juice, vinegar, salt, pepper, and caraway. Grate the fresh horseradish into it. Remove any blemishes on the beets but you don't need to peel the roots completely.
— Using a fine grater, grate the beets directly into the marinade. Now also grate the apple into it, but using a slightly coarser grater. Mix everything together and season again to taste.

▶ **Variation**
As a variation, add 200 g fresh sauerkraut to this salad.

Nutritional values per portion
180 calories / 10 g total fat / 19 g total carbohydrates / 2 g protein

Cottage Cheese Salad

An abundance of colors with lots of high-quality protein.

▶ For 2 people
Easy to prepare ⊘ 10 min.

150 g cottage cheese · **1 tbsp** white wine vinegar · **1 tbsp** olive oil · **100 g** red bell pepper · **40 g** green onions · **75 g** apple · **2 tbsp** arugula · salt/freshly ground pepper

- Put the cottage cheese in a bowl and mix with the oil and vinegar. Cut the bell pepper and green onions into thin strips and the apple into small cubes, and add to the cottage cheese.
- Finely chop the arugula and mix into the salad with the salt and pepper. If necessary, season again with salt and pepper.

Nutritional values per portion
165 calories/ 8 g total fat/ 11 g total carbohydrates/ 10 g protein

Tip

Cottage cheese salad is perfect as a filling for scooped-out tomatoes or mini cucumbers. Also tastes delicious with a boiled or baked potato.

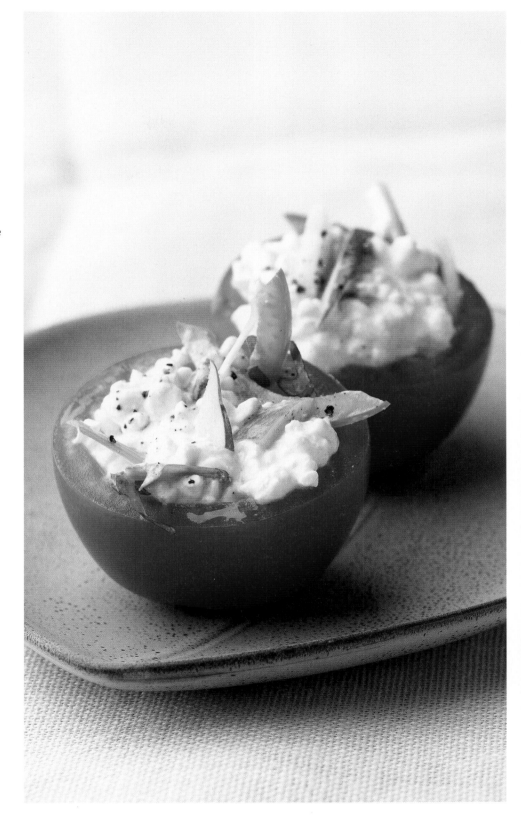

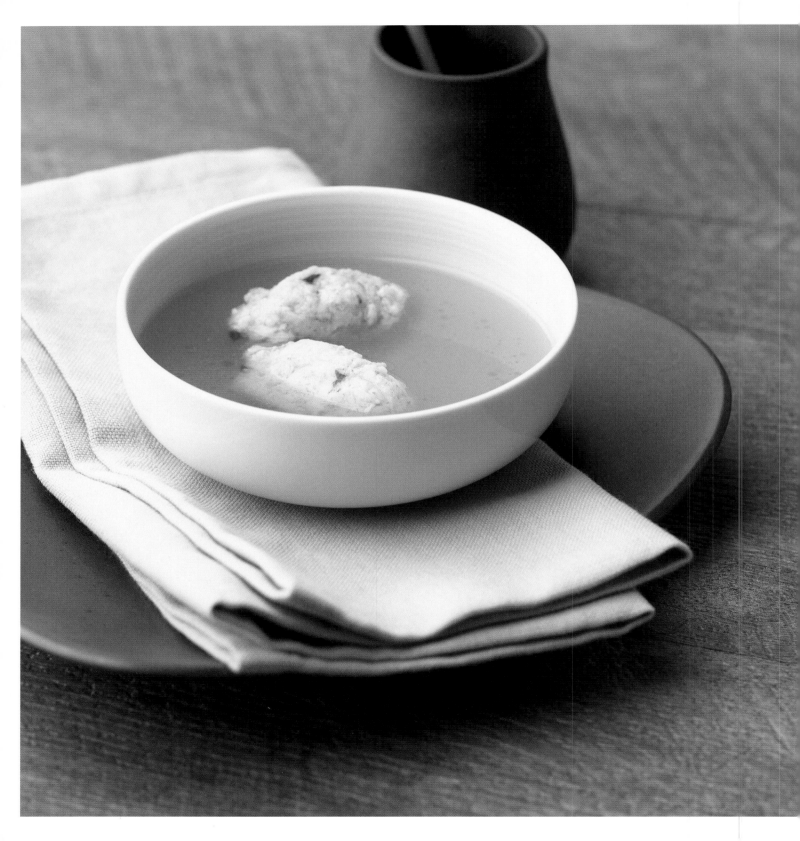

Tomato Consommé with Basil Dumplings

An elegant soup, great as an appetizer for a multi-course menu.

- Cut the onion into strips, clean the other vegetables and cut into walnut-sized cubes. Sauté with the crushed garlic. Add the tomato paste and briefly sauté a little longer. Pour in the liquid, season with salt and pepper, add the bunches of herbs, and simmer over low heat for 1 hour.
- Carefully pour the tomato stock through a fine sieve, season generously, and re-frigerate. Finely grate the clarifying vegetables, briefly beat the egg whites and add. Add everything to the cold tomato stock and return to the stove to bring to a quick boil, stirring it initially. Then let it simmer for ca. 15 min.
- Skim off the curdled egg white and vegetables and pour the remaining broth through a fine cloth. Lastly, add the balsamic vinegar.
- Coarsely grind the oats and dry-roast in a pan. Mix the quark, egg, and oats, finely mince the basil and add, then season the mixture with salt and pepper. Scoop out small dumplings and cook briefly in lightly simmering water. Serve in the soup.

▶ Info

Dry-roasting: place in a small frying pan or saucepan over a medium heat and stir for 1–2 min. until the aroma turns "nutty."

Nutritional values per recipe
425 calories / 10 g total fat / 51 g total carbohydrates / 31 g protein

Tip

If you do not own a grain mill to grind the oats, use coarse rolled oats and dry-roast them in an ungreased pan. If you want to save yourself some trouble you do not have to clarify the soup. You can simply pour the tomato stock through a fine sieve without clarifying it first.

▶ For 1.5 L soup
Requires a little more time
⊙ 30 min. + 1½ hours cooking time

For the consommé:
1 onion
200 g fresh tomatoes
50 g leek
50 g celeriac root
50 g carrots
2 garlic cloves
2 tbsp tomato paste
1.5 L vegetable broth or water
Salt/freshly ground pepper
1 bunch each of basil and rosemary

For clarifying the soup:
40 g carrots
40 g celeriac root
40 g leek (white part)
3 egg whites
1 tbsp balsamic vinegar

For the dumplings:
40 g oats
100 g skim quark
1 egg
2 tbsp basil
Salt/freshly ground pepper

Lime Soup

A very nice light dinner with some wholegrain baguette.

▶ For 1 L soup
Easy to prepare
🕐 10 min. + 15 min. cooking time
125 g leek · 125 g celeriac · 125 g fennel · 75 g parsley root · 1 L water · 2 tbsp walnut oil · salt · cayenne · a little curry powder · juice and peel from 2 limes

- Clean the vegetables and cut into walnut-sized cubes. Over medium heat, sauté until they become fragrant. Add the water and cook until the vegetables are soft.
- Put everything in a blender, add the walnut oil and spices, and purée until it is completely smooth. Gradually add the lime peel and juice. Taste the soup intermittently and stop adding lime when you have reached just the right level of tartness.

Nutritional values per recipe
315 calories/ 22 g total fat/ 22 g total carbohydrates/ 8 g protein

Chestnut Macchiato

A true feast for the eyes, served in cups or glasses.

▶ For 1 L soup
Easy to prepare
🕐 20 min. + 35 min. cooking time
50 g leek (white parts) · 50 g parsley root · 50 g parsnip · 50 g fennel · 50 g celeriac · 250 g chestnuts (can be bought pre-cooked) · 750 mL water · 250 mL soy milk (unsweetened) · salt/freshly ground pepper · 250 mL low-fat milk · 1 tsp coriander seed

- Cut the vegetables into walnut-sized cubes. Sauté over medium heat until they become fragrant. Add the chestnuts, pour in the water and soy milk, and cook until the vegetables are soft. Season with salt and pepper and purée until creamy.
- To create the foam, bring the milk with the coriander seed to a boil (low-fat milk froths particularly well) and simmer for ca. 20 min. Pour the milk through a sieve and, shortly before serving, froth it with a stick blender, whisk, or milk frother. Pour the hot chestnut soup into each cup first, then ladle the foam on top and serve immediately.

Nutritional values per recipe
820 calories/ 1 g total fat/ 11 g total carbohydrates/ 3 g protein

Creamy Beet Soup

This soup is similar to Borscht but creamier.

▶ For 1.5 L soup
Easy to prepare
🕐 10 min. + 20 min. cooking time
400 g beets · 160 g potatoes · 30 g leek · 1 tsp olive oil · 1.5 L vegetable broth · 2 bay leaves · 1 tbsp cider vinegar · 1 tsp horseradish, freshly grated · salt/freshly ground pepper

- Cut the beets and potatoes into walnut-sized cubes and the leeks into thin strips. Sauté briefly in the olive oil. Add the vegetable broth and bay leaves and simmer everything over low heat.
- Remove the bay leaves and purée the soup in a blender. Now add the cider vinegar, horseradish, and spices and season to taste.

Nutritional values per portion
75 calories/ 5 g total fat/ 5 g total carbohydrates/ 1 g protein

Asparagus Soup

A delicious variation that contains hardly any fat.

▶ For 1 L soup
Easy to prepare
🕐 10 min. + 20 min. cooking time
500 g asparagus · 3 small potatoes · ½ onion · 1 L water · a little lemon juice · salt/freshly ground pepper · 1 tbsp walnut oil · 1 tsp tarragon or dill

- Peel the asparagus and the potatoes. Cut the onions into strips and brown in a pot over medium heat. Finely chop the asparagus and potatoes, leaving the asparagus tips whole. Add everything to the pot and simmer over medium heat until it becomes fragrant.
- Add the water and cook until the vegetables are soft. Remove the asparagus tips. In a blender, combine the soup with the oil and lemon juice until it is creamy, and season to taste. Finely chop the asparagus tips and add them back into the soup. Before serving, add the minced herbs to the soup.

Nutritional values per recipe
320 calories/ 11 g total fat/ 40 g total carbohydrates/ 14 g protein

Tomato Coulis

For this dish the tomatoes should be of the highest quality.

▶ For 2 people
Budget-friendly
🕐 10 min. + 30 min. cooking time
500 g ripe tomatoes · 2 small onions 2 tbsp olive oil · 2 garlic cloves · 1 twig of rosemary

- Remove the stem end of the tomatoes and cut the tomatoes into 1-cm cubes. Finely chop the onions and brown them lightly in a little olive oil.
- Add the tomatoes and the rosemary twig, crush the garlic into the pot, and let everything simmer covered over low heat for ca. 30 min. Take out the rosemary twig, season with salt and pepper, and then add the rest of the olive oil for the final touch.

▶ Variation

Preparation is a little more involved if you peel the tomatoes beforehand. To do so, score the tomatoes with cross-shaped cuts and scald them in boiling water. Quickly rinse with cold water and peel.

Nutritional values per recipe
200 calories/ 11 g total fat/ 17 g total carbohydrates/ 6 g protein

Jerusalem Artichoke Soup

Jerusalem artichokes give the soup a wonderful creamy consistency.

▶ For 2 people
Easy to prepare
🕐 10 min. + 10 min. cooking time
100 g Jerusalem artichokes · 70 g leek · 70 g celeriac · 0.5 L vegetable broth · 50 mL milk · 1 tbsp walnut oil · salt · cayenne · a little curry powder

- Clean and finely chop the Jerusalem artichokes, leek, and celeriac. Cook the diced vegetables over medium heat in the vegetable broth until soft. Pour into the blender, add the milk and oil, purée until smooth, and season with the spices.

Nutritional values per portion
45 calories/ 3 g total fat/ 3 g total carbohydrates/ 2 g protein

Parsnip and Coconut Soup

A great warming soup for the fall or winter.

▶ For 1 L soup

Budget-friendly ⏱ 10 min. + 15 min. cooking time
200 g parsnips · **50 g** potatoes · **40 g** leek (white parts) ·
50 g grated coconut (unsweetened) · **1 L** water · **1 tbsp** walnut oil · salt · nutmeg

▬ Cut the vegetables into walnut-sized cubes. Sauté over medium heat until they become fragrant. Add the grated coconut and continue sautéing until everything is lightly browned. Add the water and cook until the vegetables are soft.

▬ Add the walnut oil and blend everything until it is very creamy. If necessary, add a little extra liquid to get the desired quantity and consistency. Season as needed and add a little ground nutmeg.

Nutritional values per recipe
565 calories/ 44 g total fat/ 35 g total carbohydrates/
8 g protein

Tip

In most cases, you won't be able to purée the grated coconut to a perfectly smooth consistency. If this bothers you, strain the soup through a sieve.

Beet Macchiato

This soup looks gorgeous served in a glass—perfect for guests.

▶ For 1 L soup

Budget-friendly ⏱ 15 min. + 30 min. cooking time
75 g potatoes · **180 g** beets · **20 g** leek · **2** bay leaves · juniper berries · **1 L** water · **1 tbsp** walnut oil · **1 tsp** cider vinegar ·
200 mL low-fat milk · **1 tbsp** freshly grated horseradish ·
1 large pinch Espelette pepper

▬ Cut the potatoes and beets into walnut-sized cubes and the leek into thin strips. Briefly brown everything together with the bay leaves and juniper berries over medium heat until it becomes fragrant. Add the water and cook until the vegetables are soft.

▬ Remove the bay leaves and juniper berries and purée the soup in the blender, adding the cider vinegar, oil, and spices and seasoning it to taste. If the soup becomes too creamy, you can adjust the consistency by adding water or vegetable broth.

▬ Simmer the milk with the horseradish and Espelette pepper for ca. 15 min., pour through a strainer, and froth with a stick blender, whisk, or milk frother. The milk should not be too hot or it will not froth well. Pour the soup into glasses, ladle the milk foam on top with a spoon and serve immediately.

Nutritional values per recipe
325 calories/ 14 g total fat/ 37 g total carbohydrates/
12 g protein

Tip

Espelette pepper is a very mild and aromatic variety of chili from France, but you can always replace this spice with a little paprika and chili powder.

▶ Beet macchiato

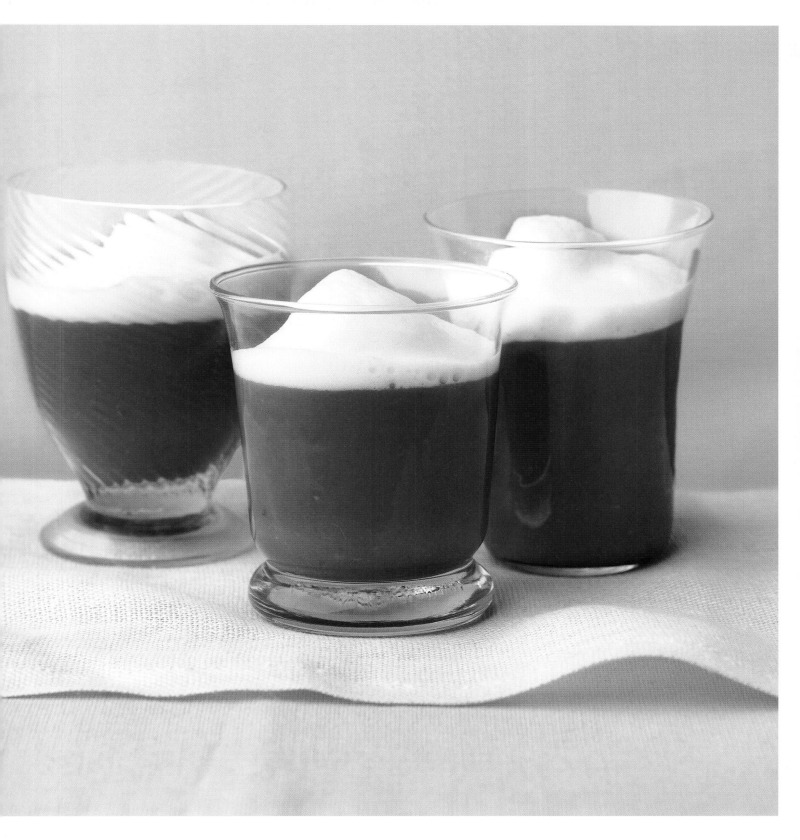

Base for Soups and Sauces

The foundation for lots of delicious soups:
with herbs and vegetables.

▶ For 1 L
Easy to prepare
⊙ 10 min. + 15 min. cooking time
300 g white vegetables (celeriac, fennel, parsley root) ·
50 g potatoes · 50 g leek (white parts) · 1 L water · 2 tbsp oil ·
salt/freshly ground pepper

━ Cut the vegetables, potatoes, and leek into walnut-sized
cubes and lightly brown over medium heat until they
become fragrant. Add the water and cook until the vegetables are soft.
━ In a blender, purée everything with whatever oil suits your
taste until very smooth. Season with salt and pepper.

Nutritional values per recipe
325 calories/ 21 g total fat/ 30 g total carbohydrates/
5 g protein

By adding various herbs and spices for flavor you can use
this base to create many different soups or sauces. In the
spring, for example, add 50 g of raw nettle tips or wild
garlic or 100 g of steamed spinach to the soup in the
blender. No doubt you can think of many other delicious
variations.

Vegetable Jus

A great base for all sorts of sauces—completely
vegetarian!

▶ For 0.5 L vegetable jus
Requires a little more time
⊙ 20 min. + 2 hours cooking time
1 carrot · ¼ celeriac · 1 medium-sized onion · 2 tomatoes ·
1 garlic clove · 1 tbsp tomato paste · 100 mL balsamic vinegar · 1 L vegetable broth · 1 twig of thyme · rosemary ·
10 juniper berries · 1 bay leaf · tamari · salt/freshly ground
pepper · 2 tbsp rice flour

━ Cut the vegetables into walnut-sized cubes and brown
briefly with the chopped garlic in an ungreased pan. Add
the tomato paste and sauté until browned. Deglaze with
the balsamic vinegar and tamari, and reduce the liquid.
Repeat this deglazing and reducing process 3 to 4 times
with the vegetable broth, then add the rest of the vegetable broth and allow it all to simmer for ca. 2 hours.
━ After half the cooking time, add the herbs and spices and
continue simmering everything. Then pour the soup
through a sieve and, if necessary, thicken with very finely
ground rice flour and season with the spices.

Nutritional values per recipe
290 calories/ 2 g total fat/ 57 g total carbohydrates/
7 g protein

You don't have to discard the vegetables afterwards,
you can purée them with vegetable broth and boiled
potatoes to create a tasty soup.

Carrot Sauce

An unobtrusive sauce that goes well with many dishes.

▶ For 1 L sauce
Budget-friendly ⊘ 10 min. + 20 min.
20 g onions · 240 g carrots · 100 g potatoes · ½ tsp turmeric ·
1 L vegetable broth or water · 1 tbsp almond oil · a small
amount of raspberry vinegar · salt/freshly ground pepper

- Cut the vegetables into walnut-sized cubes and lightly
  brown over medium heat with the turmeric until they
  become fragrant. Add the vegetable broth (or water) and
  simmer until the vegetables are soft.
- Purée everything in the blender until you have a smooth
  creamy sauce, then add the almond oil, raspberry vinegar,
  and spices, and purée everything once more. If the sauce
  is too thick you can adjust the consistency with vegetable
  broth.

Nutritional values per recipe
255 calories/ 11 g total fat/ 35 g total carbohydrates/
4 g protein

Tip

If you use curry powder instead of the turmeric the
sauce becomes spicier. A little lemongrass gives this
sauce an instant Asian touch.

Coconut Froth

A way to give local vegetables an exotic note.

▶ For 2 people
Easy to prepare ⊘ 20 min.
1 tsp ginger · 1 garlic clove · 50 g grated coconut (unsweetened) · 500 mL rice milk · lemongrass · a little Thai basil
(or lemon basil) · tamari · 2 tbsp rice flour

- Quickly sauté the ginger with the crushed garlic, add the
  grated coconut and continue cooking until lightly
  browned, then deglaze everything with the rice milk. Remove the tough outer leaves of the lemongrass stalk and
  finely dice the rest. Add to the soup, together with the Thai
  basil.
- Allow it to simmer for a while, then thicken it with the rice
  flour. Mix the stock well and strain through a sieve. Season
  to taste with a little tamari. Using a milk frother or stick
  blender, froth it into a firm foam.

Nutritional values per portion
100 calories/ 7 g total fat/ 6 g total carbohydrates/
2 g protein

Chestnut Soufflé with Grape Ragout

A delicious airy soufflé, wonderful with fully ripened grapes.

► For 2 people

Easy to prepare   ⊙ 20 min. + 30 min. baking time

200 mL vegetable broth · 1 tbsp olive oil · salt/freshly ground pepper · 50 g chestnut flour · 40 g wholegrain spelt flour · 2 eggs · ½ tsp cider vinegar · 100 g chestnuts (pre-cooked) · 200 g white grapes · 1 small red onion · 1 tbsp honey

- Bring the vegetable broth to a boil with the olive oil and a little salt. Mix the chestnut flour with the spelt flour and add all at once to the boiling liquid. Stir constantly over medium heat for 2–3 min., or until the mixture thickens and comes away from the side of the pan.
- Separate the eggs and stir the egg yolks into the slightly cooled mixture. Stir in the cider vinegar. Finely cut the cooked chestnuts and fold them in. Grease small ramekins and dust with a little flour.
- Beat the egg whites until stiff and fold into the soufflé mixture. Season well with salt and pepper and fill the ramekins with the mixture. Then bake in a 180 °C oven (160 °C convection oven) for 20 min.
- For the grape ragout, slice the grapes in half and remove the seeds. Chop the onion into thin strips. Lightly fry the onions with the honey in a pan until translucent. Briefly toss the grapes in this and arrange on a platter. Turn the soufflé out onto the grape ragout.

Nutritional values per portion

470 calories/ 13 g total fat/ 71 g total carbohydrates/ 13 g protein

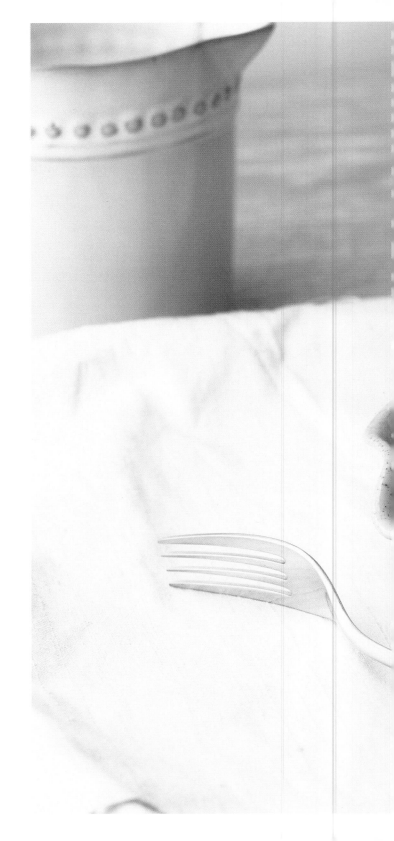

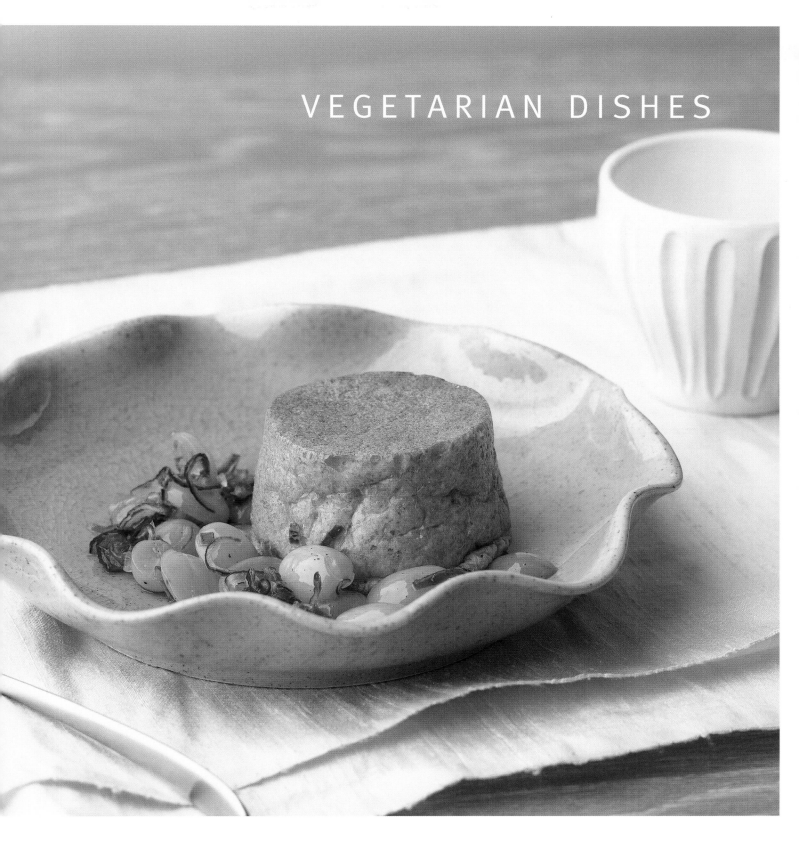

Cottage Cheese Soufflé on Vegetable Diamonds

Thanks to the cottage cheese, low in fat and high in protein.

▶ For 2 people

Easy to prepare ⊙ 40 min. + 20 min. baking time

For the cheese soufflé: 160 g cottage cheese · 160 g quark · 40 g grated Parmesan · 2 eggs · salt/freshly ground pepper · nutmeg · oil for the pan

For the vegetable diamonds: 200 g carrots · 200 g celeriac · 150 g leek · salt/freshly ground pepper · 1 tbsp olive oil · 1 tbsp minced parsley · 1 tbsp chopped chives

− For the soufflé, place the quark and cottage cheese in a fine mesh sieve and drain for ca. 30 min. Then mix the quark and cottage cheese with the remaining soufflé ingredients, stir well, and season with the spices. Lightly grease the soufflé mold and fill with the mixture. Cook the soufflé in a water bath on the stove top or in the oven, covered, for 20 min.

− For the vegetable diamonds, clean and/or peel the carrots and celeriac and cut first into 3-mm-thick slices and then into diamonds. Clean the leeks, cut in half lengthwise, then quarter, and also cut into diamonds. Sauté the vegetables over medium heat until soft.

▶ Serving suggestions

A wonderful match for the soufflé is red potato pearls: to prepare these, boil 300 g potato balls (scoop out fresh potatoes with a melon baller) in 400 mL beet juice until soft.

Nutritional values per portion
405 calories/ 21 g total fat/ 16 g total carbohydrates/ 38 g protein

Squash Soufflé

What make this dish special is that the soufflé is made with oven-roasted squash!

▶ For 2 people

Easy to prepare ⊙ 10 min. + 45 min. baking time

400 g squash · 50 g potatoes · ½ onion · ginger · curry powder · cumin · 1 egg · salt/freshly ground pepper

− Depending on the variety, peel the squash and cut into cubes. Peel the potatoes and cut into cubes as well. Chop the onion into strips. Put the vegetables in an ovenproof casserole dish, grate the ginger over them, and sprinkle with the spices. Mix everything well and bake for 20 min. in the oven at 170 °C (150 °C convection oven).

− When the vegetables are soft, remove from the oven and let them cool down a little. Now purée with the egg and again, as needed, season with the spices. Pour the puréed mixture into little soufflé dishes and bake in the oven at 160 °C (145 °C convection oven).

▶ Serving suggestions

Serve with rice noodles and coconut froth (p. 49).

Nutritional values per portion
115 calories/ 3 g total fat/ 15 g total carbohydrates/ 7 g protein

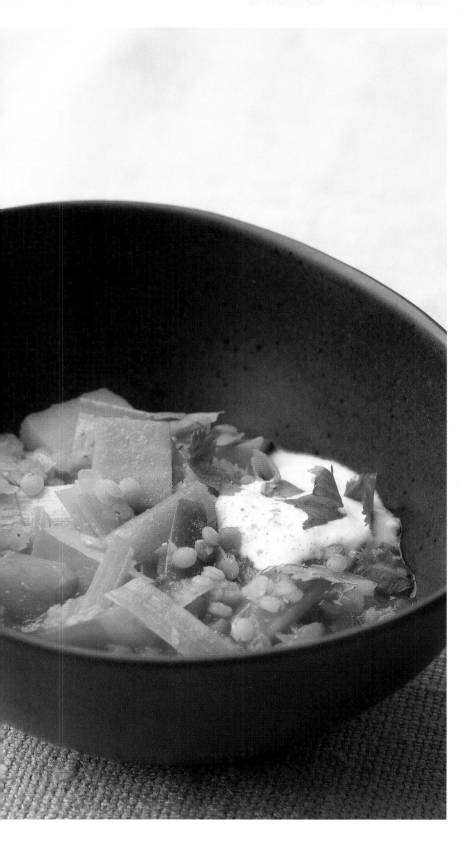

Lentil Curry

Full of spice and with an abundance
of vegetables.

▶ For 2 people
Requires a little more time
⊙ 15 min. + 45 min. cooking time
1 onion · 100 g lentils · 1 tbsp tomato paste ·
400 mL water or unsalted vegetable broth ·
1 bay leaf · 100 g carrots · 100 g leek · 100 g
squash · 100 g multicolored bell peppers ·
cumin · curry powder · chili powder · tamari ·
cider vinegar

▬ Chop the onion into small cubes and brown
lightly in an ungreased pan. Then add the
lentils and briefly sauté as well. Add the tomato paste and brown it lightly. Add the
liquid and bay leaf and cook for 30 min. until
the lentils are soft.
▬ Cut the vegetables into 1-cm cubes. Toast the
spices in a pan until they become fragrant.
Gradually add the vegetables (first the carrots, then the leeks and squash, and finally
the bell pepper), and sauté until al dente. Add
the vegetables to the lentils, let the flavors
blend for 10 min., and season strongly with
tamari and vinegar.

▶ Serving suggestions
Delicious with fresh cilantro (coriander),
yoghurt dip, and flatbread.

Nutritional values per portion
210 calories / 2 g total fat / 32 g total
carbohydrates / 15 g protein

VEGETARIAN DISHES

Fried Endives with Bulgur
A wonderful winter dish!

▶ For 2 people
Budget-friendly ⊙ 15 min. + 40 min. cooking time
2 endives · 0.5 L water · ½ tsp salt · 1 bay leaf · 1 tbsp cider vinegar · 2 tbsp wholewheat flour · 2 tsp olive oil · 40 g bulgur · 200 g carrots and celeriac · chervil · chives · salt/freshly ground pepper · 1 tsp Parmesan

▬ Put the endives in boiling water, add the bay leaf, salt, and vinegar, and simmer for ca. 30 min. Take the endives out and let them drain. Flatten gently and season with salt and pepper. Coat the endives with flour and fry on both sides in a pan with 1 tsp olive oil over medium heat until golden.
▬ Cook the bulgur in twice as much liquid until soft. Cut the carrots and celeriac into small cubes and sauté in olive oil. Add the bulgur to the sautéed vegetables and season with herbs, Parmesan, and spices.

▶ Serving suggestions
Bring 70 g Base Sauce (p. 48) to a boil, add 1 tbsp walnut oil, and round out with ½ tsp minced parsley. Pour the sauce onto the plate and place the endive on top. Press the bulgur mixture into a ladle and invert onto the plate. Sprinkle with Parmesan before serving.

Nutritional values per portion
225 calories/ 9 g total fat/ 29 g total carbohydrates/ 7 g protein

Vegetable Medley in Saffron Sauce with Rice Balls
A luscious sauce and colorful blend of vegetables.

▶ For 2 people
Easy to prepare ⊙ 10 min. + 40 min. cooking time
30 g brown rice · 1 bay leaf · unsalted vegetable broth · 2 tsp olive oil · 120 g squash · fresh ginger · curry powder · salt/freshly ground pepper · 120 g zucchini · 120 g sugar snap peas · rosemary · garlic · 60 g Base Sauce (p. 48) · 1 large pinch saffron · 1 tbsp almond oil

▬ Cook the rice with the bay leaf in 2½ times as much unsalted vegetable broth for ca. 30 min. in a covered pot until done. Before serving, season with a little olive oil and salt.
▬ Cut the squash into cubes and briefly sauté in 1 tsp olive oil. Add the finely grated ginger and season with the curry powder, salt, and pepper. Add a little broth and cook over low heat until the squash is soft.
▬ Cut the zucchinis into 0.5-cm-wide slices, cut off both ends of the snap peas and, if necessary, remove the strings. Steam the zucchinis and snap peas al dente.
▬ Toss the zucchinis with rosemary, salt, pepper, a little garlic, and olive oil in a pan. Quickly sauté the snap peas in olive oil and season with salt and pepper. Prepare the Base Sauce according to the basic recipe (p. 48). Add the saffron and stir in the almond oil. Shortly before serving, mix everything with a stick blender.
▬ Pour a glaze of sauce onto each plate, press the rice into a cup and invert it carefully onto the plate. Arrange the vegetables on top, coordinating the colors.

Nutritional values per portion
185 calories/ 8 g total fat/ 22 g total carbohydrates/ 6 g protein

Zucchini Tomato Curry with Tarragon Polenta

A true summer meal; try to prepare this recipe with fully ripened tomatoes.

▶ For 2 people
Quick to prepare   ⊘ 10 min. + 15 min. cooking time
1 onion · 1 zucchini · 2 tomatoes · 1 tsp olive oil · 1 tsp curry powder · 250 mL vegetable broth or water · salt/freshly ground pepper · 1 twig lemon balm · cumin · turmeric · 50 g polenta · 2 tbsp grated Parmesan · 1 tbsp tarragon

▬ Finely chop the onion. Cut the zucchini in half lengthwise and then into 1-cm-wide slices. Cut the tomatoes into eighths. Heat the oil, add the onion, dust with the curry powder, and sauté for ca. 3 min. Then deglaze with a little vegetable broth or water. Add the tomatoes, season, and cook covered until al dente. Pluck the lemon balm, mince it, and season the curry with it.
▬ Bring 200 mL vegetable broth to a boil and add the spices. Add the polenta to the boiling liquid and stir vigorously. Over medium heat let it simmer for 5 min. To finish, mix the Parmesan and finely chopped tarragon into the polenta and season again. With a spoon, scoop out little dumplings and arrange on a plate with the vegetable ragout.

▶ Variation
You can also cook the polenta with the same amount of beet juice. This tastes delicious and adds a beautiful dash of color.

Nutritional values per portion
145 calories/ 8 g total fat/ 13 g total carbohydrates/ 6 g protein

Black Salsify Sticks and Ragout

The sticks taste delicious with their pumpkin seed coating.

▶ For 2 people
Easy to prepare   ⊘ 10 min. + 15 min. cooking time
Juice from 1 lemon · ½ L water · 500 g black salsify · 250 mL milk (or soy milk) · 2 tbsp brown rice flour · salt/freshly ground pepper · 1 tsp almond oil · 30 g pumpkin seeds · 30 g wholewheat breadcrumbs · 1 egg · 1 tbsp wholewheat flour

▬ Add the lemon juice to the water. Peel the black salsify, cut into 5-cm pieces, and put in the lemon water until you are ready to process them further. Bring the milk to a boil, add the black salsify, and simmer until they are soft.
▬ Take out half the roots and put them aside. Sprinkle the rice flour into the milk and thicken it to a creamy consistency. Season the sauce with salt and pepper and add the almond oil for the final touch. Turn off the heat.
▬ Grind the pumpkin seeds and mix with the breadcrumbs. Whisk the egg with half the flour. Season the black salsify with salt and pepper, coat with the remaining flour, dredge in the egg-flour mixture, and lastly roll in the breadcrumbs. Fry in a lightly greased pan or drizzle with oil and bake in a 180 °C oven (160 °C convection oven) for 15 min.
▬ Reheat the ragout and serve with the black salsify sticks.

▶ Serving suggestions
Pairing this dish with the Chestnut Soufflé (p. 50) and Red Cabbage Sorbet (p. 35) turns it into a feast.

Nutritional values per portion
335 calories/ 14 g total fat/ 34 g total carbohydrates/ 20 g protein

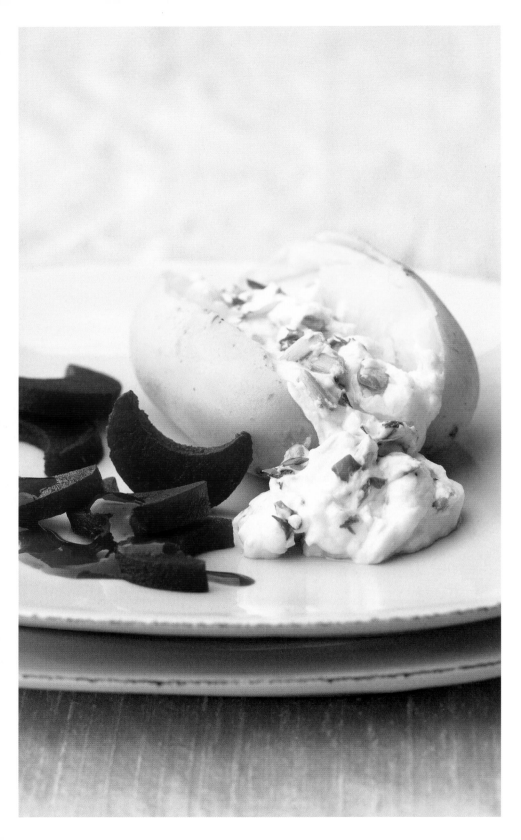

Boiled Potatoes with Budwig Crème and Beet Moons

High in protein and polyunsaturated fatty acids.

▶ **For 2 people**
Easy to prepare
⏱ **10 min. + 30 min. cooking time**
180 g potatoes · **250 g** skim quark · **2 tbsp** flaxseed oil · **2 tbsp** sunflower seeds · freshly minced herbs, e.g., dill, parsley · salt · **40 g** beets · **60 mL** beet juice · **1 tsp** brown rice flour

- Steam the potatoes.
- Using a whisk, whip the quark until smooth, add the flaxseed oil, and stir until all of the oil is emulsified.
- Roast the sunflower seeds in an ungreased pan. This gives the Budwig crème its wonderful flavor.
- Add the sunflower seeds and herbs and salt lightly. Thoroughly stir the whole mixture once more.
- Peel the beets and cut out in the shape of half moons. Cook in the beet juice until softened, and thicken with the rice flour.

Nutritional values per portion
165 calories/ 4 g total fat/ 22 g total carbohydrates/ 9 g protein

Mushroom Risotto

A great winter meal, very hearty with wholegrain risotto rice.

▶ For 2 people
Requires a little more time
⏱ 5 min. + 40 min. cooking time
100 g onions · 100 g brown risotto rice · 300 mL unsalted vegetable broth or water · 20 g dried mushrooms, e.g., porcini · 100 mL milk · 1 tsp olive oil · salt/freshly ground pepper · a little lemon juice · 200 g fresh mushrooms, e.g., oyster mushrooms · 50 g Parmesan

▬ Finely dice the onions and sauté lightly in an ungreased pan. Add the rice, toss it briefly, and deglaze with the broth. Add the dried mushrooms.
▬ Little by little, add the milk until the rice is cooked through. This takes between 30 and 40 min. Season with salt, pepper, and the lemon juice. Clean the fresh mushrooms, brown them lightly, and then add them with the Parmesan to the rice.

Nutritional values per portion
380 calories/ 13 g total fat/ 43 g total carbohydrates/ 23 g protein

Eggplants Au Gratin with Tomatoes and Mozzarella

These eggplants are particularly delightful when paired with gnocchi.

▶ For 2 people
Easy to prepare
⏱ 40 min. + 30 min. baking time
2 tbsp basil · 2 tbsp tamari · 3 tbsp water · 1 tsp olive oil · pepper · 200 g eggplant · 2 tomatoes · 1 mozzarella

▬ Pluck the basil and mix with the tamari, water, and olive oil. Cut the eggplant into 1-cm-wide slices and soak in the marinade for ca. 30 min. Cut the tomatoes into 0.5-cm-thick slices and slice the mozzarella as thinly as possible.
▬ Layer the eggplant, tomato, and mozzarella alternately in an ovenproof dish—the bottom and top layers should consist of eggplant. Cover and bake in a 160 °C oven (145 °C convection oven) for 30 min.

▶ Serving suggestions
Serve the eggplants with Tomato Coulis (p. 45), rice, bulgur, or a refreshing yoghurt dip.

Nutritional values per portion
260 calories/ 19 g total fat/ 6 g total carbohydrates/ 16 g protein

Kohlrabi Saltimbocca

A delicious vegetarian version of saltimbocca, prepared in a flash.

▶ For 2 people
Easy to prepare
⏱ 10 min. + 15 min. baking time
250 g kohlrabi · 200 g tomatoes · 10 sage leaves · 60 g mozzarella · salt/freshly ground pepper

▬ Peel the kohlrabi, cut into slices, and steam until soft. Cut the tomatoes into the same number of slices. Slice the sage leaves thinly.
▬ Arrange the kohlrabi, sage, and tomato in alternating layers in an ovenproof casserole dish and season with salt and pepper. Lastly, cube the mozzarella and sprinkle on top. Bake in a 175 °C oven (150 °C convection oven) for 15 min.

▶ Serving suggestions
Good side dishes are rice, quinoa, polenta, or wholegrain noodles.

Nutritional values per portion
130 calories/ 7 g total fat/ 8 g total carbohydrates/ 9 g protein

Napkin Dumplings with Mushroom Ragout

The extra effort is worth it. You may as well make extra dumplings—
they are also delicious fried up the next day.

► For 2 people
Requires a little more time
⏱ 40 min.
+ 45 min. cooking time

For the napkin dumplings:

300 g	stale wholewheat rolls
1	onion
1 tsp	butter
400 mL	hot milk
	Salt/freshly ground pepper
	Mace
2	eggs
2 tbsp	parsley

For the ragout:

300 g	button mushrooms (or other mushrooms)
1	onion
1	garlic clove
1 tsp	olive oil
	Thyme
200 mL	milk
1 tbsp	oat flour or other wholegrain flour
	Juice from ½ lemon
1	bunch chives

- For the napkin dumplings, cut the rolls into thin slices or cube finely. Finely chop the onion and brown in the butter. Bring the milk to a boil, season with salt, pepper, and mace, and pour this mixture over the sliced rolls. Add the onions, mix everything well, and let soak for ca. 30 min. Separate the eggs and stir the egg yolks into the bread mixture. Finely chop the parsley and add. Whip the egg whites until stiff and fold carefully into the bread mixture.
- Place a 50-cm-long strip of plastic wrap on a kitchen towel. Now spoon the dumpling mixture like a sausage into the middle of the foil. Shape the dumpling sausage into a 5-cm-thick roll, cover with the foil, and wrap in the towel. Twist the two ends of the towel in opposite directions, so that the dumpling roll becomes taut. Don't roll it too tightly, however, since the dough will expand a little. Now use string to tie the towel off like a bonbon on the right and left sides of the dough.
- In a very large pot, bring a generous amount of water to a boil. Suspend the dumpling roll in the water, securing it with the pot lid in such a way that the roll does not touch the bottom of the pot. Simmer for 30 min.
- For the ragout, cut the mushrooms into thin slices, finely dice the onion, and crush the garlic. Sauté everything together in olive oil and season with thyme and pepper. Deglaze the mushrooms with the milk and thicken with the oat flour. Season the mushrooms with lemon juice and spices. Cut the chives into little rolls and add to the mushrooms.
- Take the dumpling roll out of the water and let it rest for a moment. Untie the strings and unwrap the roll. Remove the foil. Cut the napkin dumpling into slices and serve on top of the mushroom ragout.

► Variation

The napkin dumplings are also delicious as a bread dumpling salad, made with a marinade of onions, oil, and vinegar.

Nutritional values per portion
680 calories/ 18 g total fat/ 88 g total carbohydrates/ 48 g protein

Don't add the salt to the mushrooms too early because they will absorb too much water and it will no longer be possible to brown them.

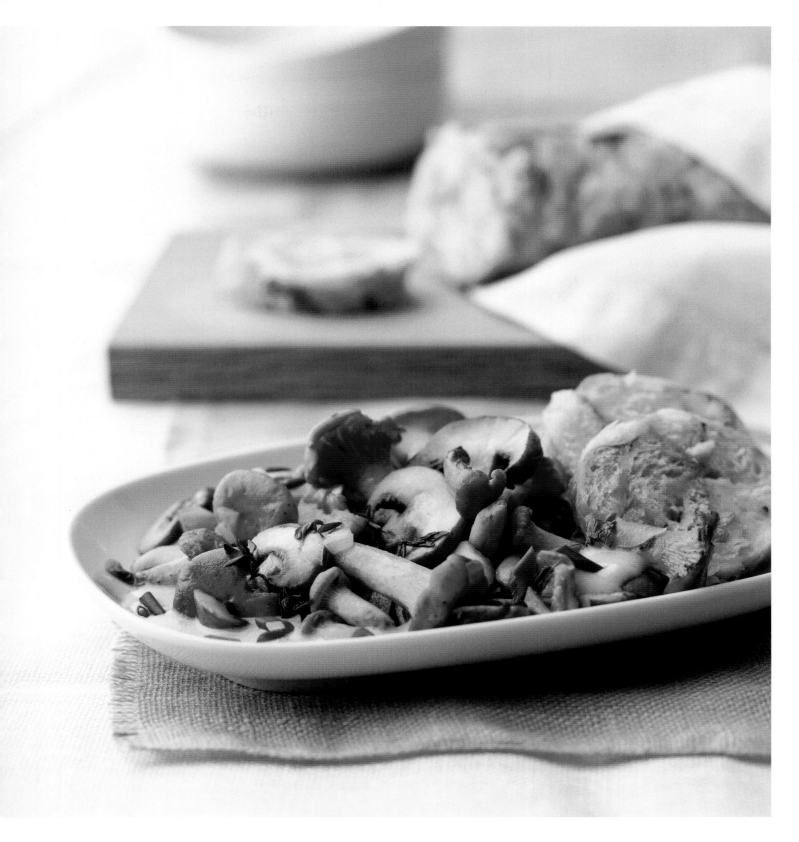

VEGETARIAN DISHES

Savoy Cabbage Roll

With a Mediterranean-style filling and very tasty!

▶ For 2 people
Easy to prepare
⊙ 20 min. + 25 min. baking time

2 large savoy cabbage leaves · 50 g red and yellow bell peppers · 100 g button mushrooms · 1 tsp olive oil · a little garlic
nutmeg · 1 twig of rosemary · salt · 100 g quark · 1 egg

▬ Wash and steam or blanch the cabbage leaves (the leaves
must be soft). Rinse briefly under cold water. Remove the
tough stems. Cut the mushrooms and bell peppers into
small cubes, briefly sauté in the oil, crush the garlic into
the mixture, and season with the spices.
▬ Drain the sautéed vegetables in a strainer. Mix the quark
and egg, add the drained vegetables, and season again.
▬ Season the cabbage with salt and pepper. Place a leaf on a
ladle, put a suitable amount of filling inside, and fold the
cabbage leaf over. Turn the two cabbage rolls over into an
ovenproof dish, add a little water, and bake in a 160 °C
oven (145 °C convection oven) for ca. 15 min.

▶ Serving suggestions
Delicious with Carrot Sauce (p. 49) and potatoes.

Nutritional values per portion
120 calories/ 6 g total fat/ 4 g total carbohydrates/
13 g protein

Potato Gnocchi

Refined with Parmesan and basil!

▶ For 2 people
Requires a little more time
⊙ 20 min. + 30 min. cooking time

For the choux dough (basic recipe): 125 mL water ·
1 tbsp olive oil · 75 g wholewheat flour · 1 egg
For the gnocchi: 300 g potatoes · 20 g Parmesan ·
1 tbsp basil · salt/freshly ground pepper

▬ Briefly bring the water and olive oil to a boil in a covered
pot. Add all the flour at once to the boiling liquid and stir
continuously. The dough will form a soft ball and pull
away from the bottom of the pot. Take the pot off the heat,
cool slightly, and then stir in the egg.
▬ Boil the potatoes in their skin, peel, and push through a
potato press. Grate the Parmesan on top and add the finely
minced basil. Knead everything into the choux dough.
Season with salt and pepper.
▬ Now roll the gnocchi dough on a smooth surface into a
1-cm-wide roll. Using a fork, lightly press a pattern into
the dough and then cut with a knife into individual gnocchi, about 2 cm long. You can now cook these in boiling salt
water or steam them.

Nutritional values per recipe
695 calories/ 24 g total fat/ 91 g total carbohydrates/
28 g protein

Tip

Depending on the season you can also use other herbs.
Squash ragout, spinach, sautéed mushrooms, or simply
a tomato sauce are excellent choices as accompanying
vegetables.

Eggplant Piccata

The vegetarian alternative to meat piccata, and very Italian!

- Pierce the eggplants with a small knife several times all over, place on a baking sheet or in an ovenproof dish and bake for 15 min. in a 160 °C oven (145 °C convection oven) until they are soft.
- Take the eggplants out of the oven and let them cool. Peel, and cut lengthwise in ca. 1-cm-wide slices. Season the eggplant slices with tamari, pepper, and rosemary.
- Whisk the eggs with 3 tbsp flour until blended. Add the milk, Parmesan, finely chopped arugula, and spices. Turn the eggplants first in 2 tbsp flour, then dip in the egg mixture.
- Put no more than 1 tbsp oil in a cold nonstick pan and drizzle ½ tsp water onto the oil. At 100 °C, the oil will start to sputter. This means that you have reached the correct temperature.
- Gently place the piccata in the pan and fry till golden yellow on both sides. If necessary, keep warm in a 160 °C oven (145 °C convection oven).

▶ Note

The correct temperature is important to prevent the egg mixture from sticking to the pan on the one hand and the piccata have a tendency to burn if the pan is too hot.

▶ Variation

This type of piccata can also be made with kohlrabi or zucchini, for example. The latter don't have to be cooked beforehand.

▶ Serving suggestions

Tomato sauce or Tomato Coulis (p. 45), served with rice, spaghetti, or polenta.

Nutritional values per portion
205 calories/ 8 g total fat/ 19 g total carbohydrates/ 13 g protein

▶ For 2 people
Requires a little more time
⊙ 25 min. + 25 min. baking time

200 g	eggplants
	Tamari
	Pepper
	Rosemary
1	egg
40 mL	milk
5 tbsp	wholewheat flour
1 tbsp	arugula
30 g	grated Parmesan
	Salt/freshly ground pepper
	Paprika
	Frying oil

Buckwheat Sauerkraut Casserole

A very hearty casserole for a healthy appetite.

▶ For 2 people
Requires a little more time
⊙ 20 min. + 80 min. cooking and baking time
100 g buckwheat · 20 g pine nuts · salt/freshly ground pepper · 1 bay leaf · parsley · marjoram · 400 g sauerkraut · 1 tsp olive oil · 20 g onions · vegetable broth · 150 g bell peppers · 30 g leek · 1 egg · 30 g cottage cheese · 30 g skim quark · 30 g feta cheese

▬ Toast the buckwheat in a 160 °C oven (145 °C convection oven) for 20 min. Then cook it in 150 mL water. The buckwheat should not be overcooked but still slightly grainy.
▬ Lightly roast the pine nuts in an ungreased pan and then mix with the buckwheat and herbs. Season with salt and pepper.
▬ Briefly sauté the sauerkraut in a little olive oil with the diced onions and the bay leaf, deglaze with a little vegetable broth, and cook until soft—this takes ca. 30 min. Cut the leek and bell peppers into strips and also sauté lightly in a little olive oil.
▬ Mix the egg with the cottage cheese, quark, and the finely cubed feta cheese. Season with salt and pepper. Mix all ingredients together and pour into a greased casserole dish. Bake everything for 30 min. in a 160 °C oven (145 °C convection oven).

Nutritional values per portion
420 calories/ 16 g total fat/ 43 g total carbohydrates/ 22 g protein

Tip
If the sauerkraut is too sour rinse it beforehand in a strainer under running water.

Spinach Polenta Gratin

This is also a great casserole to take to the office and eat cold.

▶ For 2 people
Easy to prepare
⊙ 20 min. + 35 min.
400 mL water · 1 tbsp olive oil · salt/freshly ground pepper · turmeric · cumin · 3 dried tomatoes · 100 g polenta · 1 twig of thyme · 50 g grated Parmesan · 400 g spinach · 1 onion · 1 garlic clove · nutmeg · 10 cherry tomatoes

▬ For the polenta, heat the water in a pot with the oil and spices. Finely chop the dried tomatoes and add. Stir the polenta vigorously into the boiling liquid. Simmer over low heat for ca. 5 min. Pluck the thyme and chop finely. Add half the Parmesan with the thyme to the polenta. Season again. Spread the polenta onto a lightly oiled baking sheet or in a gratin dish.
▬ For the topping, steam the spinach, rinse briefly under cold water, and chop with a knife 2 or 3 times. Finely chop the onion, crush the garlic, briefly sauté both, and add to the spinach. Season well with the spices and arrange on the polenta. Cut the cherry tomatoes in half and scatter on the gratin. Bake the gratin in a preheated 160 °C oven (145 °C convection oven) for ca. 15 min. Before serving, grate the rest of the Parmesan very finely on top.

▶ Serving suggestions
Serve with the Tomato Coulis (p. 45).

Nutritional values per portion
305 calories/ 19 g total fat/ 16 g total carbohydrates/ 15 g protein

▶ Spinach polenta gratin

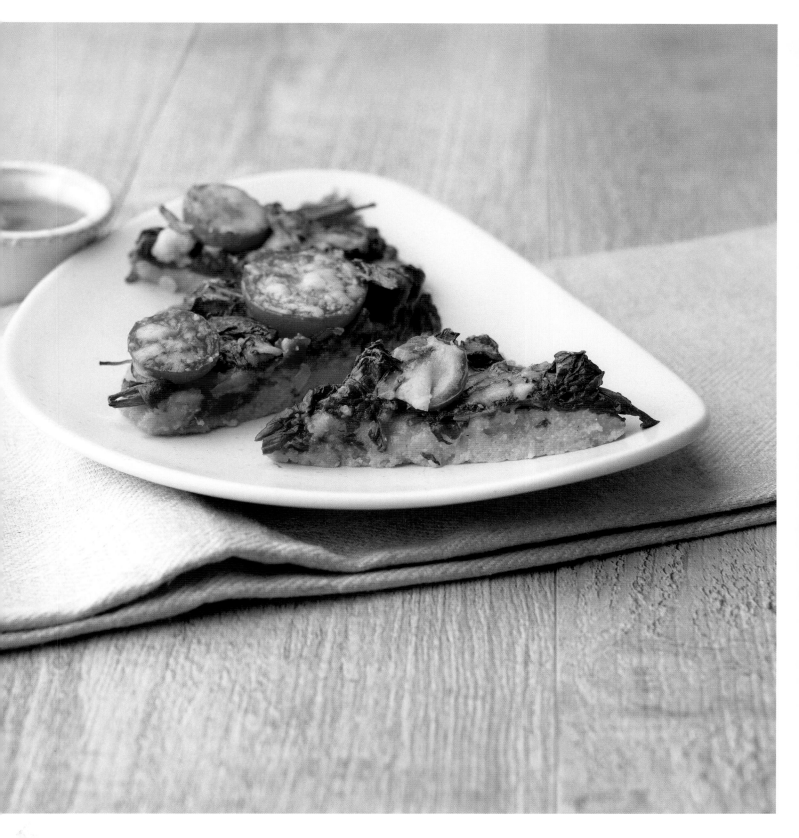

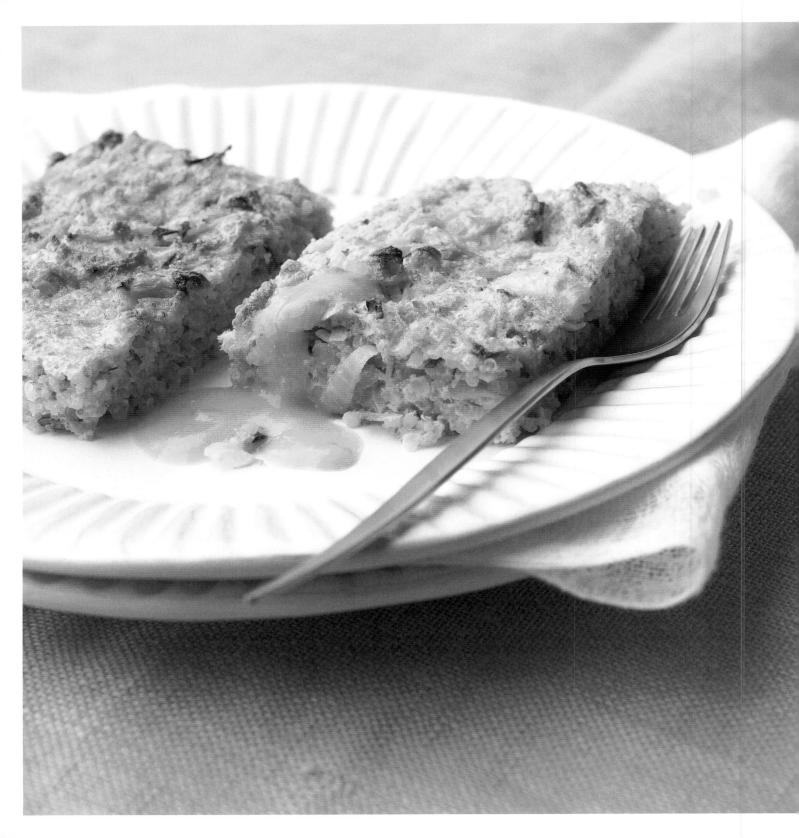

Quinoa Amaranth Casserole

In winter, simply substitute squash for the zucchini.

▶ For 2 people
Requires a little more time
🕐 20 min. + 45 min. cooking and baking time
50 g amaranth · 50 g quinoa · 200 mL vegetable broth ·
100 g carrots · 100 g zucchini · 50 g onions · olive oil · 1 garlic clove · 1 egg · 150 g quark · 40 g feta cheese · 1 bunch
chives · 40 g Parmesan, grated · salt/freshly ground pepper ·
curry powder · tamari · cayenne

▬ Rinse the amaranth and quinoa in a strainer under hot
water, dry-roast, and cook with twice the amount of vegetable broth. Coarsely grate the zucchini and carrots or cut
into thin strips. Finely dice the onions. Sauté the vegetables and onions lightly in a little olive oil, add the crushed
garlic, and cook everything until soft.
▬ Separate the egg. Blend the egg yolk with the quark until
smooth and add the finely cubed feta cheese. Mix everything with the vegetables and grains. Cut the chives into
thin rolls, beat the egg white, and gently fold both ingredients into the grain-quark-vegetable mixture. Season
with the salt, curry powder, tamari, and a little cayenne.
▬ Place the mixture into a greased casserole dish and bake
for ca. 30 min. in a 170 °C oven (150 °C convection oven).
After baking, let it rest for ca. 5 min. to make the casserole
easier to slice.

▶ Serving suggestions
This casserole tastes best with Carrot Sauce (p. 49), paired
with any vegetable in season.

Nutritional values per portion
480 calories/ 20 g total fat/ 42 g total carbohydrates/
32 g protein

◀ Quinoa amaranth casserole

Mediterranean Casserole with Feta Cheese

A light casserole with eggplant, bell pepper, and zucchini.

▶ Good for preparing ahead of time
For 2 people
🕐 10 min. + 45 min. cooking and baking time
400 g potatoes · 1 onion · 1 small eggplant · 1 zucchini ·
1 bell pepper · 1 garlic clove · 8 olives · 200 mL vegetable
broth · milk or soy milk · 2 tbsp ground oats · salt/freshly
ground pepper · thyme · 60 g feta cheese

▬ Steam the potatoes, let them cool, and peel and slice them.
Clean the onions and vegetables and cut into slices or
strips. Beginning with the onion and eggplant, lightly
sauté the vegetables. After 4 min., add the zucchini and
bell pepper, add the crushed garlic, and briefly sauté everything together with the olives.
▬ Deglaze with the liquid (vegetable broth and milk or soy
milk) and thicken with the ground oats. Mix the vegetables with the potatoes and season with the spices. Pour the
mixture into a casserole dish and crumble the feta cheese
on top. Bake the casserole for ca. 15 min. in a 180 °C oven
(160 °C convection oven).

Nutritional values per portion
335 calories/ 10 g total fat/ 45 g total carbohydrates/
14 g protein

Tip

If you don't own a grain mill just use coarse rolled oats.

FACTS

Dry-roasting

Place in a small frying pan or saucepan over a medium
heat and stir for 1–2 min. until the aroma turns "nutty."

VEGETARIAN DISHES

Swiss Chard and Mushroom Cannelloni
Quite refined, even the dough is homemade!

- For the dough, mix the olive oil, 1 large pinch of salt, and turmeric until smooth and add to the durum wheat. Now add the hot water and knead everything for ca. 5 min. Wrap in foil and allow to rest for at least 30 min. Roll the dough out thinly and cut into long strips, 10 cm wide.
- For the filling, finely dice the onions, thinly slice the mushrooms, and steam the Swiss chard briefly and then cut into thin strips. Briefly sauté the onions with the mushrooms and Swiss chard, then mix with the cottage cheese and finely chopped tomatoes. Lastly, season with a little minced arugula, salt, pepper, and nutmeg.
- Spread the filling 1 cm high on top of the dough strips, roll the cannelloni up and cut into individual pieces. Place the filled cannelloni side by side in an ovenproof dish, cover with tomato sauce, and bake in a 160 °C oven (145 °C convection oven) for 30 min.

Nutritional values per portion
335 calories/ 5 g total fat/ 48 g total carbohydrates/ 21 g protein

With the exception of the tomatoes, all the above-mentioned ingredients are available in winter. During winter use a high-quality product in a jar for the tomato sauce, or cook a tomato sauce from canned tomatoes.

▶ For 2 people
Requires a little more time
⊘ 50 min. + 30 min. baking time

For the pasta dough:
1 tbsp olive oil
1 large pinch turmeric
150 g ground wholegrain durum wheat
90 mL hot water

For the filling:
100 g onions
200 g mushrooms
200 g Swiss chard
100 g cottage cheese
2 dried tomatoes
Arugula
Salt/freshly ground pepper
Nutmeg
1 jar organic tomato sauce
(or Tomato Coulis p. 45)

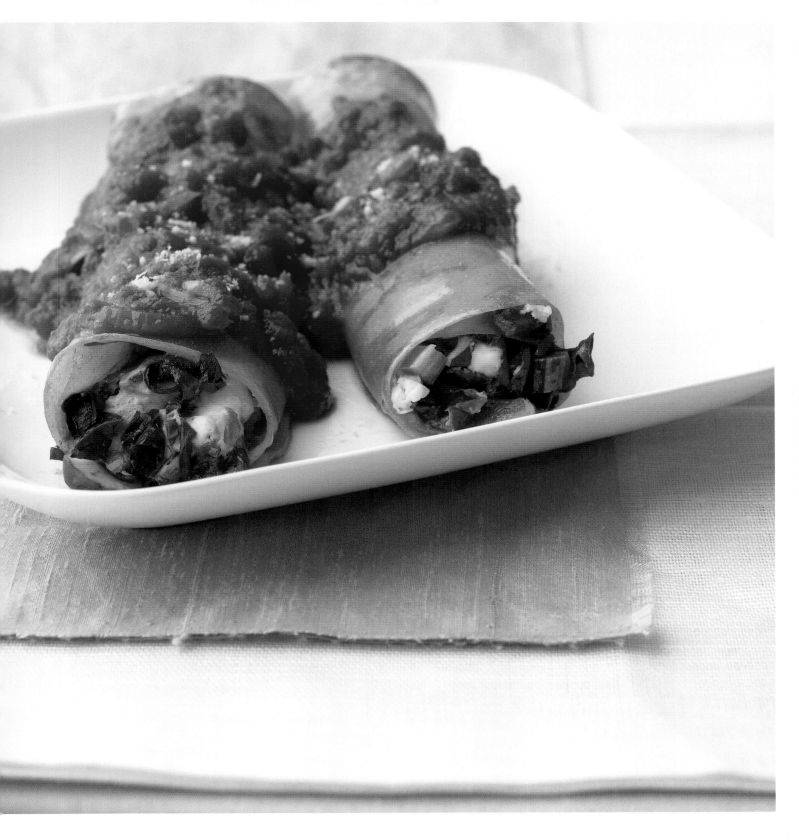

VEGETARIAN DISHES

Fennel Zucchini Lasagne with Cashew Nut Sauce
Why not prepare a large lasagne and invite friends for dinner?

▶ For 2 people
Requires a little more time
🕐 1 hour + 45 min. cooking and baking time

150 g ground wholegrain durum wheat
1 tbsp olive oil
1 large pinch turmeric
90 mL hot water
200 g fennel
Olive oil
Lemon zest
Salt/freshly ground pepper
200 g zucchini
1 garlic clove
Thyme, rosemary
100 g cashew nuts
1 L vegetable broth

■ For the pasta dough, mix the olive oil, 1 large pinch of salt, and turmeric until smooth and add to the durum wheat. Add the hot water and knead everything for 5 min. Wrap in foil and allow to rest for at least 30 min. Roll the lasagna dough out thinly and cut it in such a way that it fits into your lasagne dish.
■ For the filling, cut the fennel into slices and sauté in a pan on both sides in a little olive oil. Season the fennel with the lemon zest, salt, and pepper, add a little liquid, and cook until soft. Cut the zucchini lengthwise into slices, season with salt, pepper, and crushed garlic, and fry on both sides.
■ For the sauce, pour the hot vegetable broth over the cashew nuts, let them soak for 15 min., and then purée them. Bring everything to a boil and, if necessary, purée again.
■ Pour a little sauce into the bottom of the lasagne dish, on top of which you place the first pasta layer. Spoon the zucchini and a little sauce on the pasta layer, then add another pasta layer and spread the fennel on top of that. Drizzle with more sauce and again cover with pasta and zucchini. Cover the final layer with the sauce and bake for 30 min. in a 160 °C oven (145 °C convection oven).

▶ Variation

As an alternative to the cashew sauce, you can also prepare everything with tomato sauce or even with a basic vegetable sauce. In this case, you should, however, cover the lasagne with a little cheese and gratinate for a richer taste.

Nutritional values per portion
615 calories/ 31 g total fat/ 61 g total carbohydrates/ 23 g protein

Stuffed Portobello Mushrooms

The vegetable filling with herbs and olives turns
the mushrooms into true delicacies.

▶ For 2 people

Easy to prepare   ⊙ 20 min. + 30 min. cooking time

2–4 large portobello mushrooms · salt/freshly ground
pepper · lemon juice · 100 g tomatoes · 100 g eggplant ·
100 g zucchini · 2 olives · 50 g onions · 1 tsp olive oil ·
garlic · thyme · basil

- Wash the mushrooms, break off the stems, and season
  with salt, pepper, and a little lemon juice. Heat the pan and
  fry the mushroom caps on both sides until golden brown.
  Place the mushrooms with the stem end facing down on
  a rack to let them drain.
- Remove the peel and seed from the tomatoes. Cut the
  vegetables into 0.5-cm cubes. Finely dice the olives and
  onions. Carefully heat the olive oil in the pan and briefly
  sauté the onions. Add the olives, zucchini, and eggplant,
  and cook everything al dente.
- Lastly add the tomato cubes, toss everything briefly, and
  season with spices and herbs. Fill the mushroom caps with
  this mixture and heat for 10 min. on a baking sheet or in an
  ovenproof dish in a 160 °C oven (145 °C convection oven).

Nutritional values per portion

105 calories / 4 g total fat / 6 g total carbohydrates /
11 g protein

Tip

**Serve with risotto. If you cannot find large mushrooms,
you can of course fill a number of small ones.**

Celeriac Cordon Bleu

Delicious in the summer with a large plate of salad.

▶ For 2 people

Budget-friendly   ⊙ 10 min. + 30 min. cooking time

1 celeriac · 50 g radicchio · 40 g cheese (e.g., parmesan or
alpine cheese) · 1 tbsp tamari · 1 tbsp sesame seeds · 4 tbsp
breadcrumbs · 1 egg · a little wholewheat flour · salt/freshly
ground pepper · 1 tbsp frying oil

- Peel the celeriac and cut into 0.5-cm-thick slices. Do not
  use the end pieces, but save them for a soup or sauce base.
  Steam or cook the slices until soft. Cut the radicchio into thin
  strips, add the grated cheese, and season with the tamari.
- Mix the sesame seeds with the breadcrumbs, whisk the
  egg. Place the flour, breadcrumbs, and whisked egg separately on three plates. Season the celeriac slices with salt
  and pepper. Cover half of the slices with the radicchio-
  cheese mixture, place a matching slice of celeriac on top,
  and press down lightly.
- Turn the celeriac cordon bleu first in the flour, then in the
  egg, and then in the breadcrumbs. Press lightly at the ends.
  Sauté the cordon bleu on both sides in a pan in the oil or
  brush with the oil and bake for 15 min. in a 180 °C oven
  (160 °C convection oven).

▶ Variation

If you coat the slices separately—without any filling—with
the breadcrumbs, you get Schnitzel. You can also use
kohlrabi slices or zucchini slices, in which case you don't
have to pre-cook the zucchini.

▶ Serving suggestions

Serve with boiled or mashed potatoes, red cabbage, or
Black Salsify Sticks and Ragout (p. 55).

Nutritional values per portion

285 calories / 15 g total fat / 21 g total carbohydrates /
16 g protein

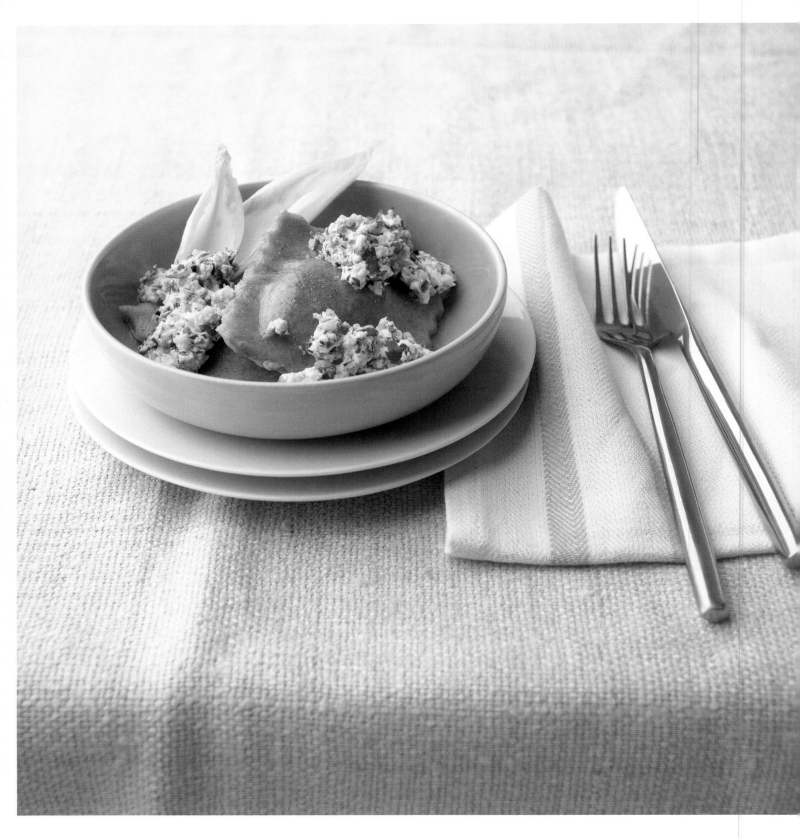

Endive Ravioli with Walnut Pesto

The effort is well worth it! For this feast invite some guests.

- For the pasta dough, stir the olive oil, salt, and turmeric until smooth and add to the durum wheat. Now add the hot water and knead everything for ca. 5 min. Wrap in foil and allow to rest for at least 30 min.
- For the filling, cut the endive and leeks into thin strips and quickly sauté with the crushed garlic in a pan. Crumble the feta cheese on top and let it melt in the pan. Season the filling with salt, pepper, and thyme.
- Roll the dough out very thinly and divide into two halves. Now place small heaps of filling onto the first sheet of dough, separated from each other by the width of the cookie cutter. Place the second sheet of dough on top, press the dough down firmly around the filling, and then cut out the ravioli. Knead the end pieces of the dough together again, roll out again, and fill.
- For the walnut pesto, finely grind the walnuts and pine nuts with a nut grinder or cheese grater. Blend with the ricotta and slowly drizzle in the oil, stirring continuously until you have achieved the desired consistency. Mince the parsley, add to the cheese and nut mixture, and season with salt and pepper.
- Cook the ravioli either in a clear vegetable broth or in salt water, or fry in olive oil without pre-cooking them (both takes ca. 4 min.).

▶ Serving suggestions
Serve with spinach.

Nutritional values per portion
700 calories/ 38 g total fat/ 58 g total carbohydrates/ 30 g protein

TIP

Ravioli is ideal for freezing. Prepare double the recipe, and you will have a little stockpile.

▶ For 2 people
Requires a little more time
⊙ 90 min.

For the pasta dough:
1 tbsp olive oil
1 large pinch salt
1 large pinch turmeric
150 g ground wholegrain durum wheat
90 mL hot water

For the filling:
150 g endive
50 g leeks
Garlic clove
50 g feta cheese
Salt/freshly ground pepper
Thyme

For the walnut pesto:
200 g walnuts
50 g pine nuts
100 g ricotta
40 mL walnut or olive oil
1 bunch parsley
Salt/freshly ground pepper

In addition: ravioli cookie cutters

Green Spelt Burgers

Prepare double or triple the quantity—these burgers also taste delicious cold.

▶ For 2 people
Easy to prepare
🕐 10 min. + 35 min. cooking time
100 g coarsely ground green spelt · 1 tbsp tomato paste · 200 mL vegetable broth (or water) · ½ onion · 1 carrot · 1 tbsp olive oil · 1 garlic clove · 1 twig of marjoram · 1 egg · salt/freshly ground pepper

- Lightly toast the green spelt in a dry pan, add the tomato paste, and deglaze with the vegetable broth. Bring to a boil and then let the grain soak up the liquid. Finely dice or grate the onion and carrot and lightly sauté in half the oil. Add the crushed garlic, and mix with the green spelt mixture.
- Pluck and mince the marjoram and add with the egg to the green spelt mixture. Season with salt and pepper. Shape the dough into small patties and fry in a pan with oil or bake in the oven.

▶ Variation
You can refine the burger mixture with a little grated cheese or mustard. Simply knead both into the green spelt dough before frying it.

Nutritional values per portion
285 calories/ 9 g total fat/ 39 g total carbohydrates/ 11 g protein

Tip

Turn the green spelt burgers into a break time snack. Take a wholewheat roll and spread with mustard, ketchup, or any of the spreads from this book. Cover with lettuce, cucumber, and tomato, and a green spelt burger. You can do the same with the Eggplant Piccata (p. 61) or the Chickpea Burgers (p. 86).

Chickpea Burgers

Very filling and high in complex carbohydrates.

▶ For 2 people
Requires a little more time
🕐 1 hour + 12 hours soaking time
100 g chickpeas · 1 bouquet garni (bay leaf, parsley, thyme) · 100 g potatoes · curry powder · cumin · 40 g carrots · salt/freshly ground pepper · nutmeg · tamari · frying oil

- Soak the chickpeas a day in advance and then cook in vegetable broth with the bouquet garni until done. Let it cool. Steam and peel the potatoes. Finely mince the chickpeas in a food processor. Press the potatoes through a potato press and mix with the chickpeas.
- Toast the curry powder and cumin in a pan until the spices become fragrant. Cut the carrots into very thin strips (julienne) and briefly sauté with the spices. Add the chickpeas and potatoes to the carrots and mix everything well. Season with nutmeg, cumin, and tamari. Shape the mixture into small burgers and fry in a little oil over medium heat until golden yellow.

▶ Serving suggestions
Delicious with a radish ragout, but also goes very well with zucchinis and eggplants. A yoghurt or tomato dip is perfect for completing the meal.

Nutritional values per portion
140 calories/ 4 g total fat/ 20 g total carbohydrates/ 5 g protein

Tip

These burgers don't hold up well when kept warm because they dry out quickly.

▶ Green spelt burgers

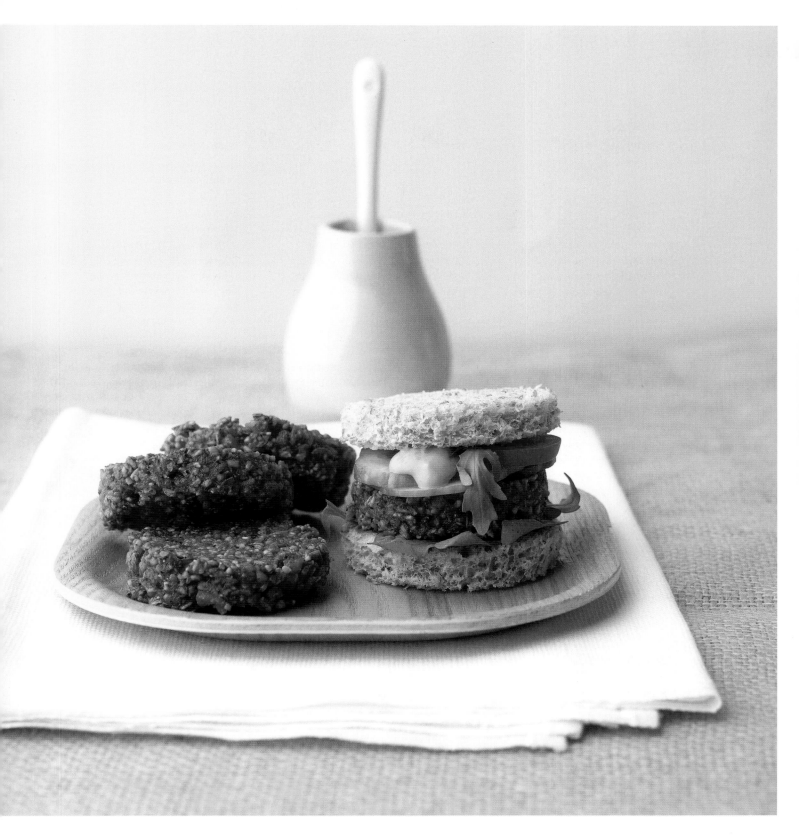

Buckwheat and Oat Burgers

With a lot of healthy fiber.

► For 3–4 people
Requires a little more time
🕐 20 min. + 35 min. cooking time
100 g buckwheat · 100 g oats ·
20 g rolled oats · 1 egg · 50 g quark ·
50 g carrots · 50 g zucchini · 20 g
grated Parmesan · 1 tsp tamari ·
1 large pinch curry powder · salt/
freshly ground pepper

– Toast the buckwheat in a dry pan
  and then cook it in twice the
  amount of water. Cook the oat
  grains in three times the amount of
  water. Finely grate the carrots and
  zucchinis and sauté briefly in a pan.
  Mix all the ingredients together and
  season heartily with the spices.
– Form into burgers and fry over
  medium heat in a little oil or bake
  for 15 min. in a 160 °C oven
  (145 °C convection oven).

► Serving suggestions
  Taste good with sautéed leek and
  a beet sauce, but these burgers are
  also delicious cold.

Nutritional values per burger
120 calories/ 3 g total fat/ 18 g
total carbohydrates/ 6 g protein

Tofu Kamut Burgers

Ingenious, with a hazelnut crust!

► For 8 burgers
Easy to prepare
🕐 10 min. + 15 min. cooking time
100 mL water · 1 tsp olive oil · salt ·
turmeric · 50 g wholegrain Kamut or
spelt flour · 1 egg · 100 g smoked
tofu · 100 g plain tofu · 1 tbsp pine
nuts · 50 g mushrooms · 20 g hazelnuts

– Bring the water to a boil with the oil
  and spices. Add the flour all at once,
  stir with a spoon, and cook for ca.
  2 min. over medium heat, stirring
  constantly. Place the dough ball in
  a bowl and use a cooking spoon or
  hand mixer to incorporate the egg.
  Finely purée the tofu and add to the
  dough. Toast the pine nuts in an
  ungreased pan, finely slice and
  brown the mushrooms. Knead
  everything together. Grind the
  hazelnuts finely.
– Shape the mixture into 8 burgers
  and turn them in the nuts to coat
  them. Fry in a small amount of oil or
  brush with oil and bake for 15 min.
  in a 170 °C oven (150 °C convection
  oven).

Nutritional values per burger
90 calories/ 5 g total fat/ 5 g total
carbohydrates/ 6 g protein

Squash Potato Pancakes

Potato pancakes with an extra dose
of beta-carotene.

► For 2 people
Easy to prepare
🕐 20 min. + 20 min. cooking time
100 g potatoes · 400 g squash · 1 egg
1 tbsp wholegrain wheat or spelt
flour · salt/freshly ground pepper ·
½ bunch chives · 1 tbsp oil

– Wash and peel the potatoes. Cut the
  squash in half, remove the seeds,
  and peel if necessary. Coarsely grate
  the squash and potatoes. Mix the
  grated vegetables with the egg,
  flour, salt, and pepper.
– Season the pancake batter with the
  chopped chives. Heat a small
  amount of oil in a pan and fry the
  pancakes in this until golden yellow.

Nutritional values per portion
190 calories/ 8 g total fat/ 20 g total
carbohydrates/ 8 g protein

► Squash potato pancakes

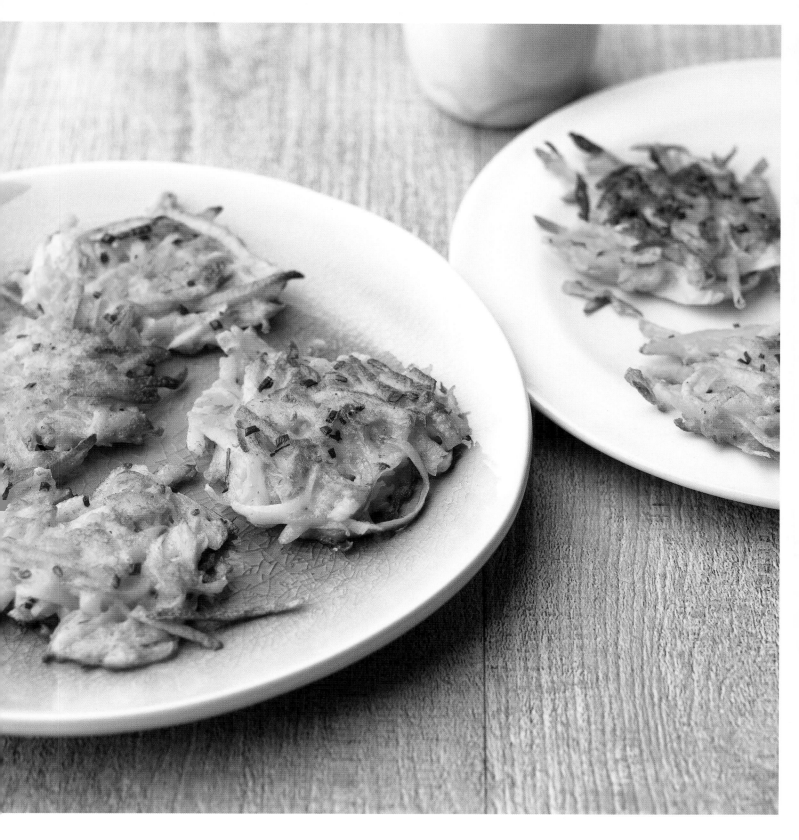

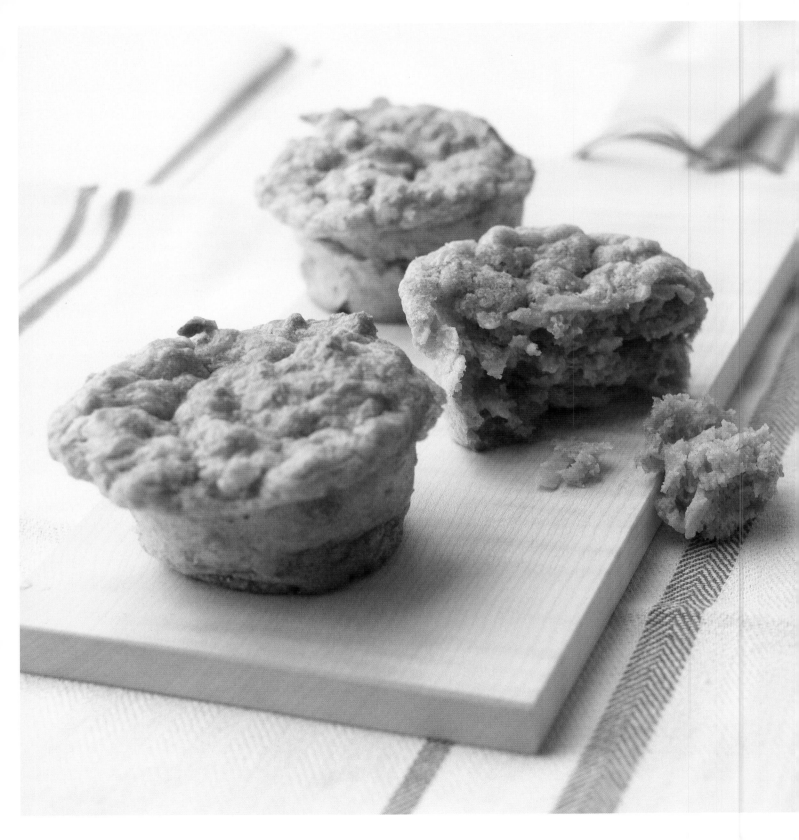

Savory Carrot Cake

This carrot cake is a wonderful choice as a slightly unusual side dish for a vegetable meal.

▶ For 1 cake
Easy to prepare
🕐 15 min. + 30 min. baking time
2 eggs · 70 g butter · 70 g quark · 200 g wholewheat flour · 200 g carrots · 1 tsp cream of tartar baking powder · 2 large pinches salt · curry powder · ginger · grated peel of 1 lemon · 140 mL milk

— Separate the eggs. Cream the butter with the egg yolks. Whip the quark separately and beat the egg whites until stiff. Stir the quark into the butter and egg mixture. Finely grate the carrots.
— Mix the dry ingredients with the carrots and the spices. Combine the dry and wet ingredients, while at the same time adding the milk, and lastly fold in the beaten egg whites. Pour into a greased cake pan and bake for ca. 30 min. at 170 °C (150 °C convection oven).

Nutritional values per cake
1500 calories / 77 g total fat / 147 g total carbohydrates / 54 g protein

◀ Savory carrot cake

Asparagus Quiche with Swiss Cheese

A little rich, but simply delicious!

▶ For 1 quiche
Good for preparing ahead of time
🕐 50 min. + 50 min. cooking and baking time
For the pastry dough: 250 g wholewheat flour · 125 g cold butter · 1 pinch salt · 3 tbsp water
For the filling: 2 kg asparagus · 300 g skim quark · 1 tbsp almond oil · 1 egg · salt/freshly ground pepper · nutmeg · 50 g Swiss cheese · 1 tbsp tarragon · olive oil

— For the dough, process the flour and butter as cold as possible. Cut the butter into small pieces, add to the flour, and work it in with 2 dough scrapers or a pastry blender, or rub it into crumbs between your hands. Make a well in the flour-butter mixture.
— Add all the other ingredients for the dough, mix well with the help of the dough scrapers, and quickly knead into a firm dough. Roll out the dough, line a baking pan with it (26–28 cm diameter), and refrigerate, covered, for ca. 30 min. Pre-bake the crust for 10 min. at 180 °C (160 °C convection oven).
— For the filling, peel and steam the asparagus (not too soft) and cut into 1-cm-long pieces. Drain the asparagus well in a sieve and put the tips aside. Blend the quark with the almond oil, egg, and spices until smooth and grate the cheese into the mixture. Mince the tarragon leaves and add to the quark mixture along with the asparagus pieces.
— Pour the filling onto the pre-baked crust and bake in a 160 °C oven (145 °C convection oven) for ca. 30 min. Right before serving, sauté the asparagus tips in a little olive oil, season lightly with salt and pepper, and serve with the quiche.

▶ Variation
Instead of quark, you can use the equivalent amount of Base Sauce (p. 48) or drained cottage cheese.

Nutritional values per quiche
2610 calories / 139 g total fat / 203 g total carbohydrates / 134 g protein

Green Asparagus, Tomato, and Arugula Tart

A beautiful summer tart that is also ideal for picnics.

▶ For 1 tart
Good for preparing ahead of time
🕐 10 min. + 35 min. cooking and baking time
For the pastry dough: 200 g wholegrain spelt flour ·
100 g quark · 2 tbsp oil · 1 egg · ½ tsp cream of tartar baking
powder · 1 pinch salt · herbs to your taste
For the filling: 2 kg green asparagus · 1 tsp olive oil · 500 g
cocktail tomatoes · 1 bunch arugula · salt/freshly ground
pepper · a small amount of lemon zest · 60 g mozzarella

- For the dough, put all the ingredients in a bowl and quickly knead to make a firm dough. Roll it out right away, place in a baking pan (28 cm in diameter), and pre-bake for 8 min. at 160 °C (145 °C convection oven).
- Remove the woody ends of the green asparagus. Cut the rest into 2-cm-long pieces. Heat the olive oil lightly in a pan, add the asparagus, and cook over medium heat.
- Cut the cocktail tomatoes into quarters, and just before the asparagus is soft, add the tomatoes, arugula, and spices to the pan. Season the vegetables, pour into the crust, and cover with the diced mozzarella. Bake the tart for 15 min. in a 170 °C oven (150 °C convection oven) until done.

Nutritional values per tart
955 calories / 40 g total fat / 74 g total carbohydrates /
71 g protein

TIP

Do not let the dough rest before baking it. Quark-oil dough toughens very quickly. After you have pre-baked it you can let it rest for several hours.

Savory Cheesecake

Combined with a fresh salad, a perfect lunch or dinner.

▶ For 1 cake
Easy to prepare
🕐 10 min. + 40 min. baking time
For the dough: 150 g wholegrain spelt flour · 75 g quark ·
2 tbsp oil · 1 egg · a little baking powder · 1 pinch of salt ·
oregano
For the filling: 600 g skim quark · 150 g strong-flavored
cheese, grated · 3 eggs · salt/freshly ground pepper ·
nutmeg · 1 bunch chives

- For the dough, put the ingredients in a bowl and quickly knead into a firm dough. Roll the dough out right away, place in a baking pan (28 cm in diameter), and pre-bake for 7 min. at 160 °C (145 °C convection oven).
- For the filling, mix the quark with the grated cheese. Separate the eggs, add the yolks to the quark, and beat the whites until stiff. Season the quark-egg mixture with the spices, cut the chives into little rolls, and carefully fold these into the quark-egg mixture, along with the whipped egg whites. Pour the filling onto the pre-baked crust and bake in a 160 °C oven (145 °C convection oven) for ca. 30 min.

Nutritional values per cake
1910 calories / 75 g total fat / 116 g total carbohydrates /
185 g protein

TIP

The cheesecake has a tendency to brown very quickly. If necessary, reduce the temperature or cover the cake.

Leek and
Swiss Cheese Tart

The tart is perfect for a buffet.

▶ For 1 tart
Good for preparing ahead of time
⊘ 20 min. + 45 min. cooking and
baking time

For the dough: 150 g wholewheat flour ·
75 g quark · **2 tbsp** oil · **1 egg** · a little
baking powder · 1 pinch of salt · oregano
For the filling: 1 kg leek · **1 tsp** olive oil ·
salt/freshly ground pepper · **3 tbsp** rice
flour · 50 g Swiss cheese

- For the dough, put the ingredients in
a bowl and briefly knead into a firm
dough. Roll the dough out right away,
place in a baking pan (28 cm in diameter), and pre-bake for 7 min. at 160 °C
(145 °C convection oven).
- For the topping, cut the leek into very
thin strips and briefly sauté in olive oil.
Season with salt and pepper and thick-
en with the rice flour. Cover the pre-
baked crust with the leek and grate the
Swiss cheese on top. Bake the tart for
ca. 30 min. in a 175 °C oven (150 °C
convection oven).

Nutritional values per tart
1380 calories / 53 g total fat / 149 g total
carbohydrates / 74 g protein

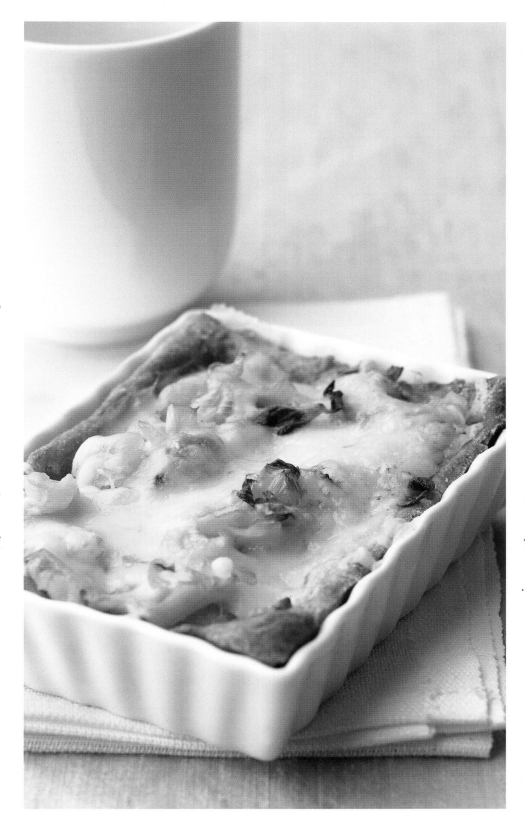

Exotic Treats

For many of the following recipes, you need ingredients that only grow in warmer or very distant regions: exotic spices, lemongrass, ginger, or special seaweed for sushi. As long as you do not use such imported products on a daily basis, you can and should enjoy them. This is a wonderful way to supplement your regional and seasonal cooking.

Winter Radish Salad with Honey

This salad is a nice complement to vegetarian sushi.

▶ For 2 people
Easy to prepare   ⊙ 15 min. + 30 min. soaking time
1 tbsp sesame oil (toasted) · 1 tbsp sesame oil (raw) · 2 tbsp
rice or cider vinegar · 1 tbsp honey · a little fresh horseradish
a little ginger · 1 stalk lemongrass or lemon rind · salt/freshly
ground pepper · 300 g black radish

– Blend the oil, vinegar, and honey. Grate the horseradish and ginger on top. Remove the tough outer leaves of the lemongrass and finely chop the rest.
– Wash the radish, remove blemishes in the peel, and grate directly into the marinade. Allow the salad to sit for ca. 30 min. and then season it.

Nutritional values per portion
175 calories/ 15 g total fat/ 8 g total carbohydrates/
2 g protein

Sweet and Sour Plum Sauce

Delicious with almost all Asian dishes.

▶ For 1 L sauce
Easy to prepare   ⊙ 10 min. + 20 min. cooking time
100 g onions · 1 chili pepper · 1 tbsp curry powder · 1 tsp
sesame oil (toasted) · 1 star anise · ½ tsp coriander seed ·
40 g ginger · 100 g prunes · 120 mL rice vinegar · 100 mL
tamari · 0.75 L prune juice

– Finely dice the onions. Seed the chili pepper and mince it. Quickly sauté the onions and chili in the sesame oil. Add the curry powder, star anise, coriander, ginger, and prunes, and sauté for 2 min.
– Now deglaze with the rice vinegar and tamari, add the prune juice, and simmer for ca. 15 min. Remove the star anise. Purée the rest with a stick blender and season well.

Nutritional values per recipe
810 calories/ 14 g total fat/ 143 g total carbohydrates/
19 g protein

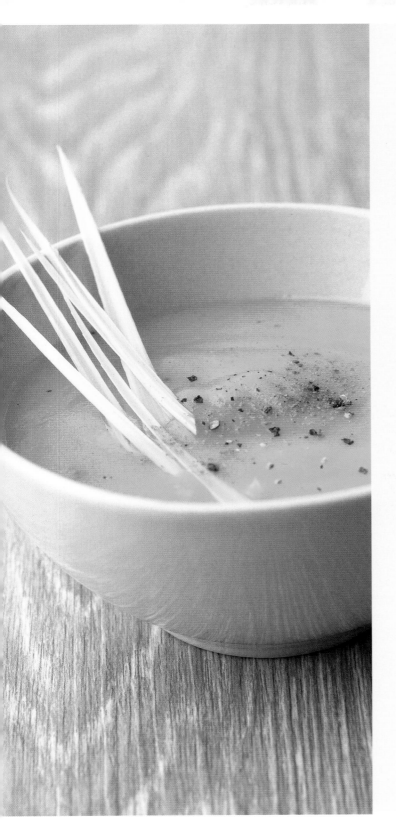

Lemongrass Squash Soup

On hot days, this soup also tastes very good cold.

▶ For 2 people

Easy to prepare   ⊙ 10 min. + 20 min. cooking time

120 g squash · 1 stalk lemongrass · 2 tbsp onions · a little ginger · curry powder · 400 mL vegetable broth or water · 1 tbsp almond oil · a little raspberry vinegar · salt/freshly ground pepper

- Cut the squash into walnut-sized cubes. Remove the tough outer leaves of the lemongrass and finely chop the rest. Finely chop the onions. Briefly sauté the onions, lemongrass, squash, and spices in an ungreased pan. Deglaze with the liquid and cook until soft.
- Purée the soup in a blender until smooth and creamy. Season with salt and pepper. Add the almond oil and raspberry vinegar and blend once more. If the soup is too thick, you can adjust the consistency by adding vegetable broth or milk.

Nutritional values per recipe

125 calories / 10 g total fat / 7 g total carbohydrates / 2 g protein

FACTS

Spices from Abroad

From the perspective of climate protection it is not necessary to give up spices from other countries or continents altogether. You may not be able to find a local source for certain spices but who would want to live without pepper or nutmeg? Transport by plane is extremely harmful for the climate, several hundred times more damaging than transport by ship. It is therefore better to steer clear of goods transported by plane. Nevertheless, spices are generally transported worldwide by ship and some "exotic" spices are even grown domestically, so we do not have to give up tamari, cumin, saffron, or turmeric. Pleasure and climate protection are therefore not mutually exclusive.

Satay Sauce

Great with spring rolls or spicy marinated chicken skewers.

▶ For 2 people
Good for preparing ahead of time
🕒 10 min. + 20 min. cooking time
30 g onions · 1 garlic clove · 1 tsp sesame oil (toasted) · a little ginger · curry powder · cumin · 500 mL vegetable broth · 50 g unsalted peanuts · 100 mL coconut milk · 1 tbsp rice flour · 2 tbsp tamari

▬ Dice the onions, crush the garlic, and briefly sauté both in the sesame oil. Finely grate the ginger and add, sprinkle the curry powder and cumin on top, and deglaze with the vegetable broth.
▬ Chop the peanuts, dry-roast them, and add to the broth. Stir in the rice flour and add the tamari. Reduce everything down to a third, add the coconut milk, bring to a boil, and purée in the blender to create a light creamy sauce.

Nutritional values per recipe
415 calories/ 31 g total fat/ 17 g total carbohydrates/ 17 g protein

Tip

You can also make your own coconut milk. Simply bring 1 part grated coconut and 2 parts water to a boil and let it soak for 2 hours.

Squash Balls

A great vegetable dish to accompany Indian curries.

▶ For 2 people
Easy to prepare
🕒 20 min. + 20 min. cooking time
300 g Hokkaido squash · ½ onion · 1 tbsp squash seeds · a little ginger · 2 tbsp olive oil · 50 mL vegetable broth · 1 tbsp grated coconut · 2 dried figs · ½ tsp lemongrass · 1 tbsp tamari

▬ Carve balls out of the squash with a melon baller or cube the squash into 1-cm pieces. Peel and cube the onion. Lightly toast the squash seeds in an ungreased pan. Add the onion and the squash balls, grate the ginger on top, drizzle with the oil, and cook over medium heat.
▬ Bring the vegetable broth to a boil with the grated coconut, strain, and add to the squash. Cut the dried figs into fine cubes and add to the squash, along with the lemongrass. Cook until done. Lastly add the tamari and season to taste.

Nutritional values per portion
215 calories/ 16 g total fat/ 12 g total carbohydrates/ 5 g protein

Spring Rolls

An Asian appetizer, delicious with the Satay Sauce (p. 82).

▶ For 2 people
Easy to prepare
🕒 20 min. + 25 min. cooking and baking time
100 g cauliflower florets · 100 g sugar snap peas · 100 g spring onions · 100 g Chinese cabbage · 100 g oyster mushrooms · 100 g mung bean sprouts · curry powder · cumin · ginger · 1 tbsp sesame · 1 tbsp rice flour tamari · 4 sheets spring roll wrappers or rice paper · 1 tsp sesame oil

▬ Cut the vegetables into thin strips. Heat the curry powder, ginger, and cumin in a pan until the spices are fragrant. Add the vegetables and sauté briefly. Toast the sesame seeds and add to the vegetables.
▬ Lastly, add the rice flour. This is done to thicken the extra liquid and prevent the spring rolls from getting soggy. Season the vegetables with the tamari and spices.
▬ Distribute the vegetable mixture on the spring roll wrappers, roll them up, and place on a greased baking sheet. Spray the spring rolls with sesame oil and bake for 15 min. in a 180 °C oven (160 °C convection oven).

Nutritional values per portion
270 calories/ 8 g total fat/ 37 g total carbohydrates/ 12 g protein

Asian Beansprout Stir-fry

A colorful stir-fry with tofu and cashew nuts.

▶ For 2 people
Easy to prepare   ⊙ 20 min. + 30 min. cooking time
1 garlic clove · 1 small onion · ½ tsp ginger · ½ tsp curry powder · chili powder · ½ tsp cumin · 200 g tofu · 50 g carrots · 50 g kohlrabi · 50 g shiitake or oyster mushrooms · 50 g zucchini · 50 g multicolored bell peppers · 50 g snap peas · 120 g mung or soy bean sprouts · 1 tbsp sesame oil (toasted) 1 tbsp honey · 200 g vegetable broth · 2 tbsp rice flour · tamari · 1 tbsp fresh cilantro · 20 g cashew nuts (toasted)

- Crush the garlic, finely chop the onion and ginger, and put everything in a pan with the curry powder, cumin, and chili. Heat carefully. Cut the tofu into 1-cm-thick cubes, add and brown. If necessary, add a little sesame oil.
- Cut the vegetables into small slivers of equal length and add gradually as appropriate for their cooking time. Cook until soft. First add the carrots and kohlrabi, then the mushrooms, then the other vegetables, and at the very end the sprouts, heating them only briefly.
- Deglaze everything with the vegetable broth, sprinkle in the rice flour, and bring to a quick boil. Season with the tamari and remaining sesame oil. Mince the cilantro and add it together with the toasted cashew nuts.

▶ Serving suggestions
Rice or rice noodles go very well with this dish. But it can also be paired nicely with the Satay Sauce (p. 82).

Nutritional values per portion
375 calories/ 17 g total fat/ 32 g total carbohydrates/ 25 g protein

Tip

When toasting the spices, don't let them get too hot because they tend to burn quickly and taste bitter.

Japanese Vegetable Stir-fry with Coconut Froth

Delicious with buckwheat noodles.

▶ For 2 people
Easy to prepare   ⊙ 20 min. + 30 min. cooking time
For the stir-fry: 150 g shiitake mushrooms · 150 g red onions 150 g red bell pepper · 150 g Swiss chard (with stem) · 1 tbsp sesame seeds · curry powder · cumin · garlic · ginger · 1 tbsp sesame oil · tamari
For the coconut froth: 1 tsp ginger · 1 garlic clove · 50 g grated coconut · 500 mL rice milk · lemongrass · a little Thai basil (or lemon basil) · 2 tbsp rice flour

- Cut the mushrooms into strips, the red onions into narrow wedges, and the bell pepper into long strips. Separate the Swiss chard stems from the green leaves and cut into long strips. Cut the leaves in half lengthwise and also cut into strips.
- In a pan, heat the sesame seeds with the ginger, garlic, onions, curry powder, and cumin until they become fragrant. Then add the vegetables and sesame oil. As the last step, add the Swiss chard leaves and sauté briefly. Deglaze with the tamari and season with the same spices that you already used above.
- For the coconut froth, briefly sauté the ginger with the crushed garlic, add the grated coconut and brown lightly, then deglaze with the rice milk. Remove the tough outer leaves of the lemongrass and finely dice the rest. Add to the coconut, together with the Thai basil.
- Allow it to simmer for a while, then thicken with the rice flour. Mix well and strain through a sieve. Season to taste with a little tamari. Using a milk frother or stick blender, froth it into a stiff foam.

▶ Serving suggestions
Serve with buckwheat noodles. You can also pair this dish with roasted poultry.

Nutritional values per portion
390 calories/ 22 g total fat/ 33 g total carbohydrates/ 17 g protein

Vegetarian Sushi

Here is proof: sushi is also great without fish.

▶ For 12 nori sheets
Good for preparing ahead of time
⏲ 40 min. + cooling and
marinating time

For the rice:
500 g brown short-grain rice
1.4 L water
60 mL rice vinegar
¼ tsp salt

For the filling:
Hoshinori or Yakinori seaweed
sheets
Wasabi horseradish
Avocado
Cucumber
Radish
Carrot
Tofu
Mushrooms
Freshly grated ginger
Garlic
Lemongrass
Tamari
Curry powder
Cumin
Miso paste
Toasted sesame oil

In addition:
Bamboo mat (for rolling sushi,
can be found in Asian markets)
Pickled ginger
Tamari

- Wash the rice, let it drain, and cook until soft in 1.4 L water. When the rice is done, stir in the rice vinegar and salt. Let the rice cool before you continue with the recipe.
- For the filling, quickly sauté the tofu and mushrooms, finely grate the carrot and radish. Cut the avocado into long strips. Peel the cucumber and cut into strips. Marinate the vegetables and tofu: suitable spices include ginger, garlic, lemongrass, tamari, curry powder, cumin, miso paste, and toasted sesame oil.
- Place a sheet of nori on the bamboo mat, spread a very thin layer of wasabi on it (it is very hot), and cover two-thirds of it with a 0.5-cm-thick layer of sushi rice. Leave a 1-cm-wide strip empty along the upper edge. Place the filling on that. Now roll up the bamboo mat, beginning from the lower edge.
- Be careful that the nori sheets do not break and that you form a nice firm roll. Remove the bamboo mat and cut the roll into pieces with a sharp kitchen knife that has been dipped in cold water. Serve with a little sweet-and-sour pickled ginger and wasabi. To dip the sushi, prepare a small dish with tamari or serve with the Plum Sauce (p. 80).

Nutritional values per roll
115 calories / 2 g total fat / 17 g total carbohydrates / 7 g protein

FACTS

Rice for sushi

For sushi it is really important that the rice is cooked correctly. To get a sticky consistency, use brown short-grain rice. With brown rice you can only add salt or acids after it is cooked because these prevent the rice from softening.

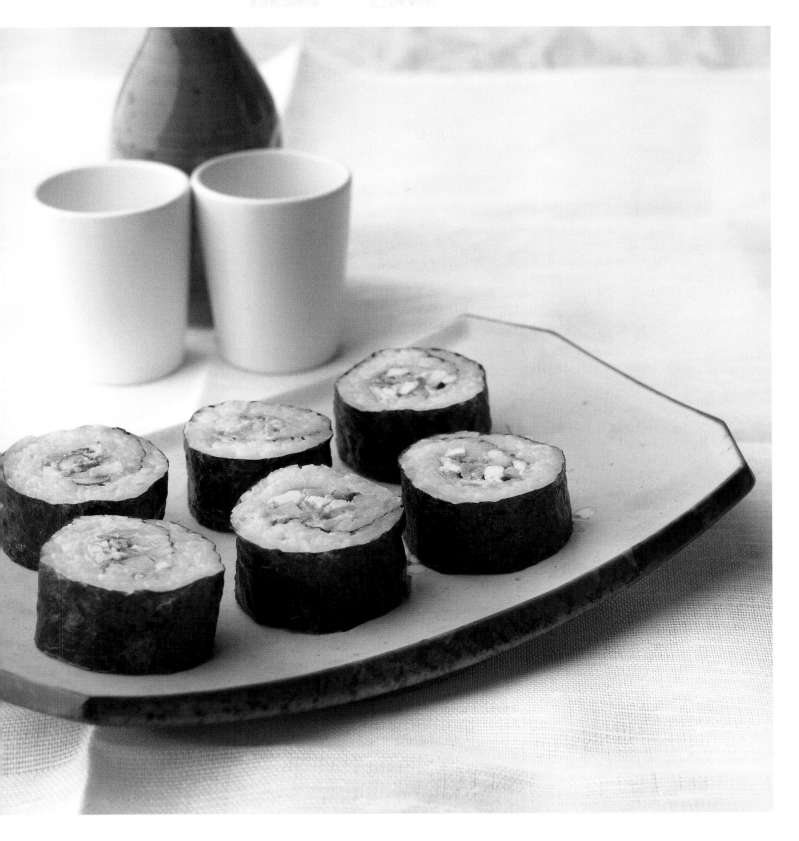

Braised Rabbit

In case you have never dared to cook rabbit before,
the preparation is easy.

▶ For 6 people
Requires a little more time
⏱ 20 min. + 1½ hours cooking time
1 rabbit (2–2.5 kg) · 1 tbsp frying oil · salt/freshly ground
pepper · 1 onion · 1 carrot · 1 leek · 1 small celeriac ·
1 tbsp tomato paste · 0.25 L red wine

— Separate the shoulders and legs from the trunk of the rabbit. Cut the back fillets off the bone, trim the meat neatly, and refrigerate. Cut the shoulders, legs, breast flap, and neck into larger pieces and season strongly with salt and pepper.
— In a casserole, strongly brown the meat pieces all over in a little frying oil. Cut the vegetables into walnut-sized pieces, add to the meat, and sauté quickly. Add the tomato paste and sauté some more until everything is browned. Then deglaze with the red wine. Add 250 mL water and braise in a 140 °C oven (125 °C convection oven) for 1¼ hours. If necessary, add a little water now and then.
— Remove the rabbit pieces and keep warm. Reduce the sauce to 250 mL, pour through a strainer, and season again. Brown the back fillets in a hot pan with a little frying oil and let them cook for 5 minutes. Return the meat pieces to the sauce, reheat, and serve arranged with the carved back fillets.

▶ Serving suggestions
Serve with mashed potatoes or Jerusalem artichokes.

Nutritional values per 100 g
160 calories/ 7 g total fat/ 1 g total carbohydrates/
20 g protein

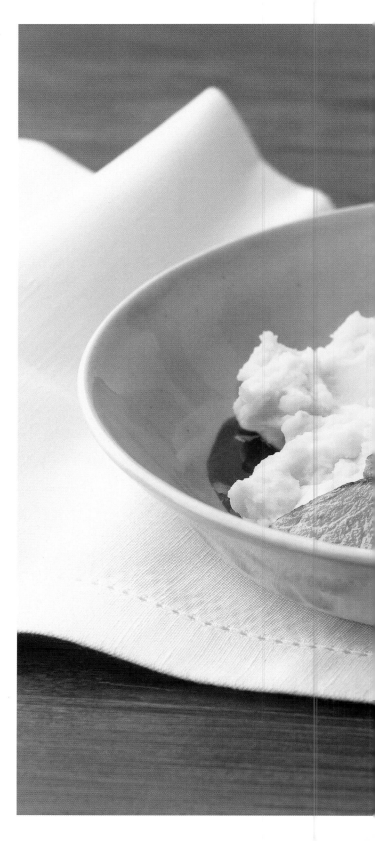

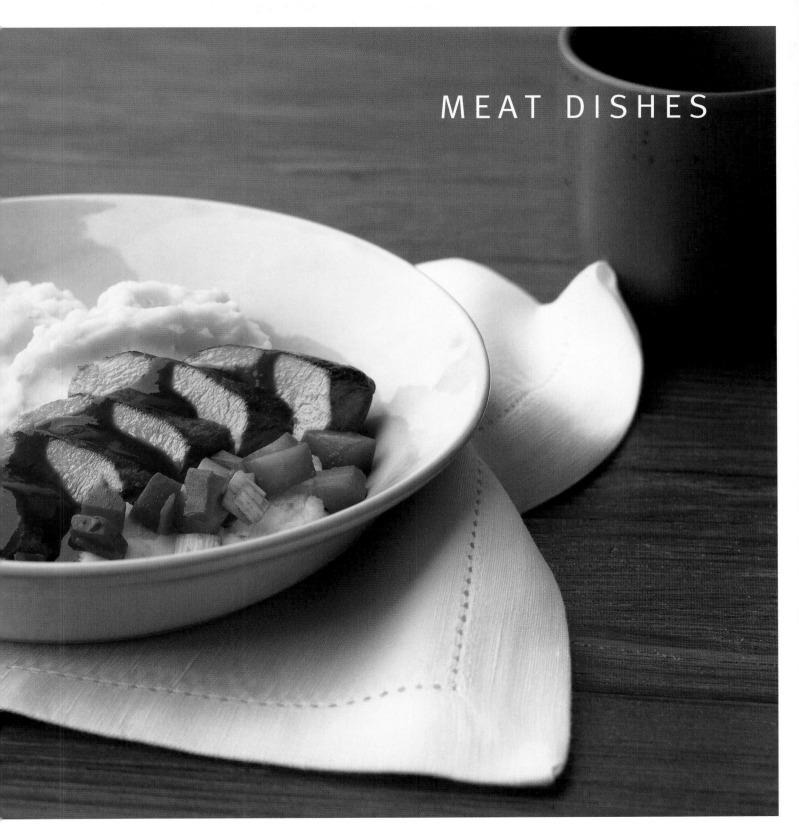

MEAT DISHES

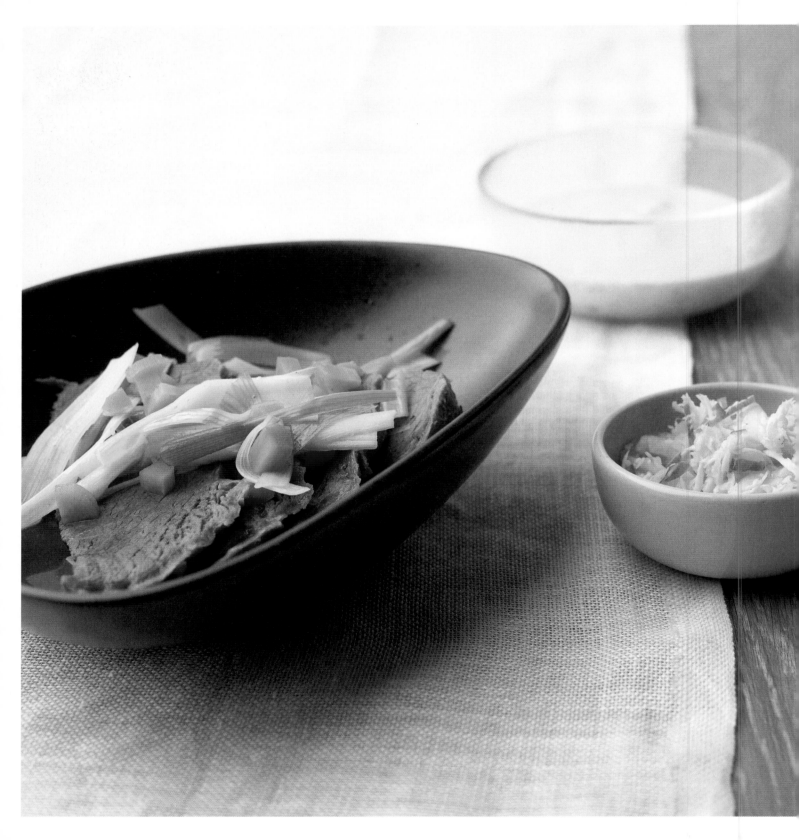

Boiled Beef with Apple Horseradish Sauce or Horseradish Bread Sauce

A classic dish with two different sauces.

▶ For 6 people
Requires a little more time
🕐 30 min. + 2½ hours cooking time
2 onions · 3 L water · salt · 2 bay leaves · 1 tsp crushed peppercorns · 2 juniper berries · a few celery greens · 1 parsley stem · 1.5 kg cap of rump (prime boiling beef) · 1 leek · 1 celeriac · 1 carrot

▬ Cut an onion in half and brown in an ungreased pot. Then add the water and bring to a boil. Add ½ tsp salt, bay leaves, peppercorns, and juniper berries. Tie the parsley stem and celery greens together and add that as well.

▬ Put the meat into the boiling water and lower the temperature so that it is only simmering gently. Cover the pot and let the meat simmer for approximately 2 hours, while regularly skimming off the foam that forms on top.

▬ Wash and peel the vegetables. Cut into cherry-sized pieces and add to the pot. Simmer everything for another 30 min. When done, remove the vegetables and meat from the broth, let the meat rest for a moment, then cut it into slices as thick as a finger. Serve together with the vegetables, covered with a little broth.

Nutritional values per 100 g
170 calories/ 10 g total fat/ 1 g total carbohydrates/ 21 g protein

---

FACTS

Horseradish

Once you have added horseradish to a sauce, do not boil it again because this will cause the mustard oils to evaporate and the sauce to lose its flavor and potentially turn bitter.

Apple Horseradish Sauce

Nice and sour, also a good accompaniment for cold roasts.

▶ For 6 people
Quick to prepare 🕐 10 min.
2 sour apples · 2 tbsp horseradish, freshly grated · a little lemon juice

▬ Cut the apples into quarters, remove the seeds, and grate finely. Mix with the horseradish and season with a little lemon juice.

Nutritional values per recipe
135 calories/ 0 g total fat/ 35 g total carbohydrates/ 1 g protein

Horseradish Bread Sauce

A creamy sauce to go with boiled beef.

▶ For 6 people
Easy to prepare 🕐 20 min.
120 g white bread, without the crust (or 3 stale rolls) · 0.25 L broth from the boiled beef · 0.25 L heavy cream · lemon juice · 3 tbsp horseradish, freshly grated · salt/freshly ground pepper

▬ Remove the crust, cut the bread finely, pour hot beef broth over it and bring to a brief boil. Add half the cream and purée this. Whip the rest of the cream and stir with the horseradish into the sauce while it is still hot. Season with lemon juice, salt, and pepper. Serve right away.

Nutritional values per recipe
1070 calories/ 81 g total fat/ 71 g total carbohydrates/ 17 g protein

Stuffed Breast of Veal

A delicious classic, perfect for a Sunday roast!

▶ For 6 people
Good for preparing ahead of time
⊘ 30 min. + 2 hours roasting time

1.5 kg	breast of veal
4	dry wholegrain rolls
1	onion
1	bunch parsley
250 mL	milk
4	eggs
200 g	veal sausage (ordered from the butcher), or Napkin Dumpling mass (p. 58) Salt/freshly ground pepper Nutmeg
1 tsp	cooking oil
200 g	veal bones
1 tbsp	tomato paste
1	carrot
1	celeriac
1	onion

- Remove any remaining gristle and fat from the veal breast prepared by the butcher. Put the veal breast aside. Cut the rolls into thin slices and finely dice the onion. Finely chop the parsley and combine all these ingredients in a bowl. Bring the milk to a boil and pour over this mixture.
- Cover and let it soak, then knead it thoroughly by hand. Add the eggs and veal sausage, process everything into an even mixture, and season with salt, pepper, and nutmeg. Spread the filling out in the center of the breast of veal and fold the ends of the meat on top of each other. Using a thread and meat needle, sew the breast together on the three open ends.
- Thoroughly brown the breast all over in a casserole with a little oil, add the bones, and place in a 140 °C oven (125 °C convection oven). Peel the vegetables and cut into walnut-sized cubes. Add to the breast after half an hour and roast with the breast, then add the tomato paste and, when everything is browned, deglaze with 750 mL water.
- The breast of veal should be done after 2 hours. Remove from the oven, reduce the sauce to 0.5 L, and purée any remaining vegetables with a stick blender. The vegetables are used here to thicken the sauce. Cut the breast into finger-width slices and remove the thread and bones before serving.

▶ Serving suggestions
Delicious with Napkin Dumplings (p. 58) and vegetables.

Nutritional values per 100 g
140 calories/ 8 g total fat/ 5 g total carbohydrates/ 11 g protein

Oxtail Ragout

A lavish dish with a great red wine sauce and wonderfully tender meat.

- Without peeling them, cut the onions, celeriac, and carrots into walnut-sized pieces. Turn the oxtail and shank slices in flour and brown in a casserole on all sides until they have turned an even light brown color. Remove both, then sauté the cut vegetables over medium heat until they are lightly browned.
- Add the tomato paste and stir. As soon as it begins to brown on the bottom of the pot, deglaze with a little balsamic vinegar and immediately afterwards with water. Let the liquid evaporate until everything starts roasting again. The vegetables should turn a nice dark color and give off an enticing roasting fragrance.
- Repeat this process 3–4 times, sprinkle 4 tbsp flour on top, then add the oxtail and veal shank slices back in, and pour the beef broth and wine on top. Add the peppercorns, juniper berries, and bay leaves.
- Roast the oxtail ragout in a 150 °C oven (135 °C convection oven) covered for 3 hours. Alternatively, you can also simmer the meat very gently in a pot on the stove (2–3 hours).
- Season the sauce with salt and a little balsamic vinegar. If you want to, remove the chunks of meat from the sauce, strain the sauce through a sieve, and add it back to the meat.

▶ Serving suggestions

Tastes delicious with Spinach Polenta Gratin (p. 62) or Puréed Beans (p. 27).

Nutritional values per 100 g
160 calories/ 11 g total fat/ 1 g total carbohydrates/ 13 g protein

▶ For 6 –8 people
Requires a little more time
⊙ 30 min. + 3 hours roasting time

3	large onions
1	small celeriac
2	medium-sized carrots
2.5 kg	oxtail (cut up)
2	crosscut slices of veal shank (ossobuco) of ca. 200 –250 g each
	Flour
2 tbsp	cooking oil
3 tbsp	tomato paste
5 tbsp	balsamic vinegar
0.5 L	water
3	bay leaves
5	juniper berries
0.5 L	dry red wine
2 L	beef broth (or water)
1 tsp	crushed peppercorns

Chicken Soup

A warming dish for cold days!

▶ For 6–8 people
Good for preparing ahead of time
🕓 20 min. + 90 min. cooking time
1 soup chicken (2.5 kg) · 1 tsp peppercorns · 2 bay leaves ·
1 small piece of ginger · 2 cloves garlic · 1 small fresh chili
pepper (medium hot) · 1 leek · 1 medium-sized celeriac ·
1 carrot · parsley stalks

— Rinse the chicken thoroughly under running water, cut off
  the fat glands. Put the chicken in a large pot and cover with
  cold water. Crush the peppercorns and add to the chicken,
  together with the bay leaves. Finely slice the ginger and
  garlic and add; also add the whole chili pepper.
— Slice the leek and carrot in half lengthwise, quarter the
  celeriac. Tie half the vegetables and the parsley stalks in a
  bundle and add to the pot. Bring everything to a boil and
  adjust the heat so that the soup is simmering gently.
  Repeatedly skim off the foam that forms on the surface.
  Cut the remaining vegetables into thin strips.
— After 1½ hours, remove the chicken from the stock, let it
  cool off a little, and take the meat off the bones. Set aside
  the breast meat as well as the meat from the drumsticks.
  If you want to, you can save this meat to make a Chicken
  Ragout (p. 94). Otherwise cut the meat from the breast and
  drumsticks into strips and set aside together with all the
  other meat.
— Pour the stock through a sieve and season with salt. Add
  the vegetable strips to the broth, wait a while, and then
  add the meat.

Nutritional values per 100 g
220 calories / 15 g total fat / 1 g total carbohydrates /
21 g protein

Rooster with Autumn Vegetables

Tender juicy meat, crispy skin, delicious vegetables from
the oven!

▶ For 6 people
Easy to prepare   🕓 20 min. + 1 hour roasting time
1 rooster (2.5–3 kg) · salt/freshly ground pepper · 3 onions ·
3 red bell peppers · 1 Hokkaido squash · lemon thyme

— Cut the rooster in half and then into pieces. Season with
  salt and pepper, set aside the breasts, and brown the rest
  of the meat in a casserole. Bake for ca. 1 hour in a 140 °C
  oven (125 °C convection oven).
— Cut the vegetables into larger chunks and add to the casserole after half an hour, along with the breast meat. Turn
  the meat repeatedly and drizzle with any fat that has ac-
  cumulated on the bottom of the pan. After about 1 hour,
  test to see if the drumsticks are soft and the vegetables
  done.
— For the last 5 min., turn on the broiler or change the oven
  setting to top heat, in order to lightly crisp the skin of the
  rooster. Pluck the leaves off the lemon thyme and sprinkle
  over the dish.

▶ Serving suggestions
Serve the rooster simply with fresh bread.

Nutritional values per 100 g
100 calories / 5 g total fat / 2 g total carbohydrates /
12 g protein

▶ Rooster with autumn vegetables

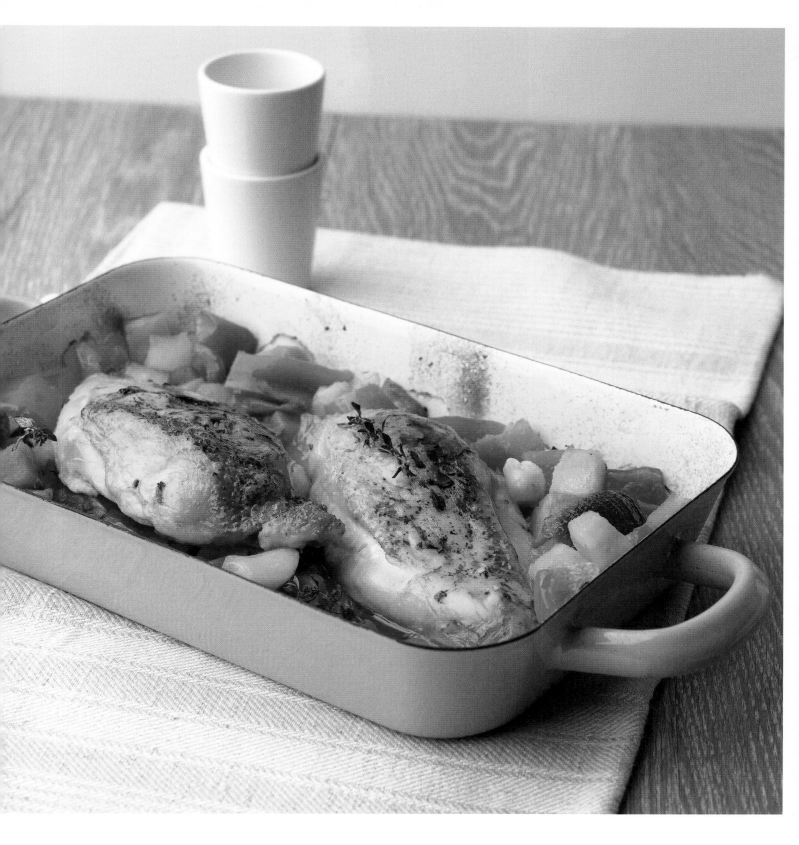

Chicken Ragout

Perfect when you have meat left over from the chicken soup.

▶ For 6 people

Quick to prepare ⊙ 20 min. + 30 min. cooking time

Meat from the breast and drumsticks of a soup chicken ·
150 g potatoes · ½ celeriac · 1 white onion · 1 leek (white
parts) · 1 medium-sized Jerusalem artichoke or parsley root ·
1 tbsp olive oil · 1 L chicken broth · 100 mL soy milk (or
cream or low-fat milk) · salt · juice from ½ lemon · 1 tbsp
tarragon · 2 tbsp chervil

— Peel the potatoes, celeriac, and Jerusalem artichoke and
  cut into walnut-sized pieces. Chop the onions coarsely into
  cubes. Cut the leek in half lengthwise and chop coarsely.
  Briefly sauté the cubed vegetables in the olive oil without
  browning them.
— Add the chicken broth to the pan and bring to a boil. Lower
  the heat and let it simmer for ca. 30 min. until the vegetables are soft. Mix with the soy milk to create a smooth
  sauce. Pour into a pot and season with salt and lemon
  juice. Cut the meat from the breast and drumsticks into
  strips and add to the sauce. Finely chop the tarragon and
  chervil and mix into the sauce shortly before serving.

▶ Serving suggestions

Serve with rice or wide noodles.

Nutritional values per 100 g
50 calories/ 3 g total fat/ 3 g total carbohydrates/ 3 g protein

Veal Heart and Tongue in a Chive Cream Sauce

An old almost forgotten recipe for Sundays.

▶ For 6 people

Easy to prepare ⊙ 30 min. + 1 hour cooking time

1 veal heart (800 g) · 1 veal tongue (800 g) · 3 L water ·
1 onion · 2 bay leaves · 4 cloves · 3 tbsp cider vinegar
For the sauce: 300 g white vegetables (celeriac, fennel,
parsley root) · 50 g potatoes · 50 g leek (white parts) ·
125 mL white wine · salt/freshly ground pepper ·
125 mL heavy cream · 2 bunches chives

— Cut the veal heart in half. Rinse the heart and tongue under
  cold running water. Put 3 L water in a pot together with salt,
  the heart, and the tongue. Cut the onion in half and stud
  with 1 bay leaf and 2 cloves each. Add this and the vinegar to
  the water. Bring to a boil, if necessary remove any foam from
  the top, and let it simmer over gentle heat.
— The tongue will be soft after ca. 45 min., the heart requires
  a little more time. Remove the tongue from the pot, let it
  cool off a little, and peel off the skin with a sharp knife.
  When the heart is soft, also remove it from the cooking
  liquid and set it aside.
— For the sauce, cut the white vegetables, peeled potatoes,
  and leek into walnut-sized cubes and sauté over medium
  heat until they become fragrant. Deglaze with the wine.
— Pour the cooking liquid through a sieve and add ca. 500 mL
  of it to the vegetables. Allow this to cook until the vegetables are soft. Add the cream, purée everything, and season
  with salt and pepper. Cut the tongue and heart into finger-
  width slices and reheat in the sauce together with the
  freshly chopped chives.

▶ Serving suggestions

Wide noodles or rice are delicious with this dish.

Nutritional values per 100 g
140 calories/ 7 g total fat/ 6 g total carbohydrates/
12 g protein

Sauerbraten from Lamb

A really special treat, the sauce is simply magnificent.

▶ For 6 people
Requires a little more time
⊘ 2 hours + 5 days marinating time

1 onion · 1 carrot · 0.25 L red wine · 0.25 L water · 2 bay leaves · 5 cloves · 10 juniper berries · 2 lamb necks (deboned), 800 g with the bones (have the butcher include them) · 1 tbsp unrefined cane sugar · salt · 1 tsp oil · 1 tbsp tomato paste · 2 tbsp wholewheat flour

▬ Cut the onion and carrot into walnut-sized cubes and put in a large bowl. Add the red wine and water as well as the herbs and spices, sugar, and a little salt. Let the meat and bones sit in this marinade for ca. 5 days. Keep in the fridge and turn repeatedly.

▬ Remove the lamb necks and bones from the marinade and dry with paper towels. Heat the oil in a casserole and brown the meat and bones all over.

▬ Take out the meat, add the tomato paste to the bones, brown it, dust with flour, and deglaze with a little marinade. Let this cook down and deglaze it again with marinade. Repeat this process until everything has turned a light brown color. Then add the meat back in. Pour the remaining marinade over everything and roast for ca. 1½ hours in a 120 °C oven (110 °C convection oven).

▬ Take out the meat, cut into finger-width slices, pour the sauce through a sieve, and it with serve the meat.

▶ Serving suggestions
Very tasty with Napkin Dumplings (p. 58) or Spinach Polenta Gratin (p. 62).

Nutritional values per 100 g
150 calories/ 9 g total fat/ 3 g total carbohydrates/ 11 g protein

Involtini

A quick Mediterranean recipe for roulades.

▶ For 2 people
Quick to prepare
⊘ 10 min. + 15 min. cooking time

For the roulades: 140 g gammon (pork ham, the muscles from the top of the inside of the leg, cut into 2 thin cutlets) · 1 small zucchini · 1 tomato · 6 basil leaves · 80 g mozzarella · 1 small onion · 3 tomatoes · 1 tsp frying oil · 1 garlic clove · 2 rosemary twigs · 1 tbsp olive oil · salt/freshly ground pepper

▬ Flatten the cutlets and season with salt and pepper. Cut the zucchini lengthwise into very thin slices, cut the tomatoes and mozzarella into thin slices, cut the basil into strips.

▬ Cover the cutlets with the zucchini and tomato slices, the basil, and lastly the mozzarella in thin layers, season with salt and pepper, and gently roll them up, securing them with a toothpick.

▬ Cube the onion and tomatoes. Add the frying oil to the pan and brown the roulades in this on all sides. Add the onions and tomatoes, as well as the crushed garlic.

▬ Season with salt and pepper, add the rosemary twigs, cover with a lid, and let the cutlets simmer for 10 min. over medium heat. Remove the rosemary before serving and drizzle with olive oil.

▶ Serving suggestions
Simply cook spaghetti, mix with the tomato sauce, and eat with the roulades.

Nutritional values per 100 g
83 calories/ 5 g total fat/ 2.1 g total carbohydrates/ 7.1 g protein

Beef "Geschnetzeltes"

The vegetables are already part of this dish.

▶ For 2 people

Easy to prepare 🕑 15 min. + 25 min. cooking time

150 g green beans · 200 g beef round (the top of the inside of the hind leg, ideal for stir-frying) · 1 tsp frying oil · 200 g multicolored bell peppers · 100 g onions · 1 garlic clove · 2 bay leaves · 1 tbsp mustard · 1 tbsp rice flour · 300 mL low-fat milk · salt/freshly ground pepper · 1 tbsp savory · 1 tbsp olive oil

- Steam the beans in a steaming basket until done, then rinse briefly under cold water.
- Slice the beef finely into strips. Cut the onions and bell pepper into very thin strips as well. Heat the frying oil in a large pan, add the beef, and brown over high heat for ca. 1 min. Add the onions, bell pepper, and bay leaves, crush the garlic into the pan, and sauté everything together for ca. 5 min.
- Cut the beans into bite-sized pieces and add to the meat, together with the mustard. Stir briefly. Dust everything with the rice flour, deglaze with the milk, bring to a boil, and season with salt and pepper. Chop the savory and add to the dish together with the olive oil.

Nutritional values per 100 g

70 calories/ 3 g total fat/ 4 g total carbohydrates/ 6 g protein

Tip

Ask your butcher what cut is most suitable for stir-frying. For example, the shank (leg of the cow), after the tendons are removed, is wonderful and much cheaper compared with the short loin or fillet. The top round or sirloin are ideal for this dish as well.

Chicken and Vegetable Stir-fry

Here, the chicken is prepared Asian-style for a change.

▶ For 2 people

Easy to prepare 🕑 15 min. + 25 min. cooking time

2 chicken drumsticks · 1 small onion · 1 carrot · 1 Jerusalem artichoke · 2 Swiss chard leaves · 1 tbsp honey · curry powder · coriander · 100 mL soy milk · 1 tbsp rice flour · salt/ freshly ground pepper

- Debone the chicken meat and slice very thinly.
- Cut the onion into strips and fry briefly in a pan over medium heat with the curry powder and coriander. When everything becomes fragrant, add the meat and turn the heat up to high. As soon as the meat is seared crispy, add the honey and caramelize it lightly.
- Cut the carrot and Jerusalem artichoke into thin slices as well, add, and stir-fry with everything else.
- Now add the chard stems, chopped into small pieces, to the pan. Shortly before the vegetables are soft, add the chopped leaves.
- Deglaze with the soy milk, thicken with the rice flour, and let it simmer for 2 minutes. Season with salt and pepper.

▶ Serving suggestions

Serve with rice or noodles.

Nutritional values per 100 g

358 calories/ 0.65 g total fat/ 79.6 g total carbohydrates/ 7.2 g protein

Pork on Lentils

A typical Sunday meal from the region of Baden in the southwest of Germany.

- Put the meat in a large pot, cover with cold water, and bring to a boil. Cook at 90 °C for 1½ hours until done. Soak the lentils for 1 hour in cold water.
- Clean the vegetables and cut into small cubes. Add the vegetable trimmings to the pork cooking liquid. Fry the onions in walnut oil until translucent. Add the celeriac and carrot cubes and season with salt and 1 pinch of unrefined cane sugar. Sauté everything together once more over high heat, add a little vegetable broth, and simmer until soft.
- Cover the lentils just barely with water and boil for ca. 15 min. until soft. When the lentils and vegetables are firm to the bite, combine and maybe add a little of the lentil cooking liquid.
- Remove the pork shoulder from the cooking liquid, let it rest a moment, and cut into finger-width slices. Arrange with the lentils and vegetables on a platter.

Nutritional values per 100 g
130 calories/ 8 g total fat/ 5 g total carbohydrates/ 10 g protein

TIP

There is an old variety of lentils that has been recultivated in the Swabian Alps, called Alb-Leisa. They taste delicious with this dish. Serve with a slice of rustic wholegrain bread and you've got the perfect meal.

▶ For 8–10 people
Easy to prepare
🕐 1 hour + 1½ hours cooking time

1	pork shoulder, pickled and lightly smoked (2.5–3 kg)
300 g	lentils
500 g	carrots
500 g	celeriac
200 g	onions
2 tbsp	walnut oil
0.25 L	vegetable broth
1	pinch unrefined cane sugar

Roasted Pike

Roasted whole and therefore nice and juicy.

▶ For 5 people
Quick to prepare
🕐 5 min. + 15 min. roasting time
1 pike (freshwater, 1.5 kg) · salt/ freshly ground pepper · juice from 1 lemon · 2 tbsp wholewheat flour · 1 tbsp roasting oil

━ Clean the pike and rinse the inside thoroughly with water. Then pat it dry with paper towels, season with salt and pepper, drizzle with lemon juice, and turn in the flour. Heat the oil in a casserole, briefly brown the pike on both sides, and continue baking for 15 min. in a 150°C oven (135°C convection oven) until done.

▶ Serving suggestions
Serve pike with oven-roasted potatoes, spinach leaves, and, if you like, with a saffron sauce.

Nutritional values per portion
280 calories/ 5 g total fat/ 3 g total carbohydrates/ 56 g protein

Steelhead Trout Tartare with Fried Quail Egg

A truly sumptuous appetizer!

▶ For 2 people
Quick to prepare
🕐 10 min. + 5 min. cooking time
200 g steelhead trout fillet · 2 tsp olive oil · 2 tbsp lemon juice · salt/ freshly ground pepper · ½ red onion · 1 tsp olive oil · 2 quail eggs

━ Cut the trout into small cubes, so finely you are almost shaving it. Marinate in 1 tsp olive oil, the lemon juice, and the seasonings. Dice the onion very finely and combine gently with the tartare.
━ Slowly heat 1 tsp olive oil in a pan with a little water. When the water begins to splatter, crack the small quail eggs carefully directly into the pan and cook over medium heat to make fried eggs. Arrange the tartare artistically on 2 plates—best done by means of a ring—and place the fried eggs on top.

▶ Serving suggestions
Tastes excellent with asparagus.

Nutritional values per portion
180 calories/ 9 g total fat/ 2 g total carbohydrates/ 21 g protein

Fish Grilled on a Salt Crust

Here you don't grill the fish inside a salt crust, but on top of it.

▶ For 2 people
Easy to prepare
🕐 40 min. + 10 min. cooking time
2 whitefish or other freshwater fish (each ca. 150 g) · 1 kg sea salt · 1 tbsp water · 2 bay leaves · 1 tbsp walnut oil · juice of 1 lemon · pepper, freshly ground

━ Cover a barbecue rack or griddle with aluminum foil. Mix the salt with the water, spread on the aluminum foil on the grill, and heat it.
━ Clean the fish under running water and place a bay leaf inside each fish. As soon as the salt has turned into a hot crust (takes ca. half an hour), dry the fish off with paper towels and place on the salt crust. After ca. 5 min. flip the fish over for the first time and then grill depending on size until the spine in the abdominal cavity has turned grey.
━ To serve, simply drizzle with the oil and lemon juice, sprinkle with pepper, and enjoy.

Nutritional values per portion
225 calories/ 11 g total fat/ 0 g total carbohydrates/ 31 g protein

Zander En Papillote

Quickly prepared, and the oven does all the work.

▶ For 2 people
Quick to prepare
⊘ 10 min. + 15 min. baking time
200 g fillet of zander · 1 carrot · ½ leek ·
½ celeriac · salt/freshly ground pepper ·
1 orange · 1 lemon · 2 sheets parchment
paper

- Divide the zander fillet into 2 pieces of equal size. Grate or cut the vegetables into very fine strips, season with salt and pepper, and mix. Arrange the vegetables in the middle of the parchment paper, season the fish and place on top of the vegetables.
- Grate a little lemon or orange zest on top. Fold the ends of the paper over the fish on top of each other and twist them together like a bonbon. Place the whole package on a baking sheet and bake in a 150 °C oven (135 °C convection oven) for 15 min.

Nutritional values per portion
120 calories/ 1 g total fat/ 7 g total
carbohydrates/ 20 g protein

FACTS

"En Papillote"

To cook dishes "en papillote," you wrap all ingredients in parchment paper and close the package up so that the fish, meat, or vegetables cook in their own juice.

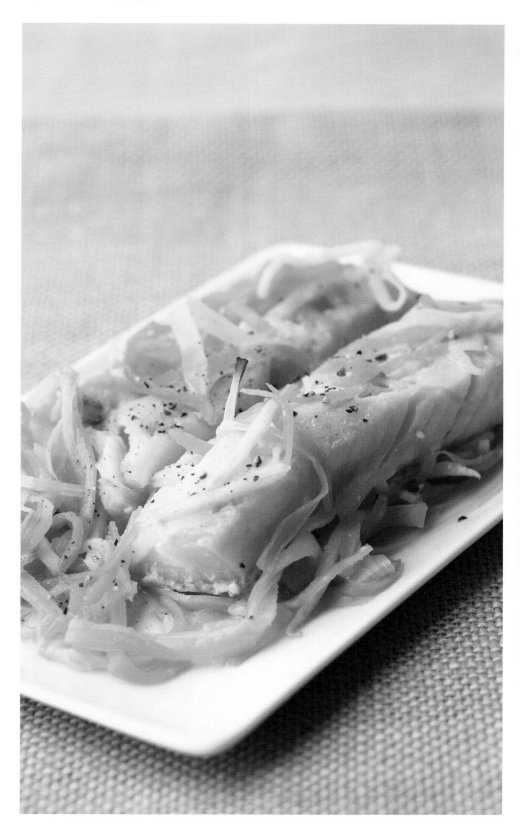

Lavender Crème Brulée

A variation on this classic dish that is low in fat and eggs, but because of the lavender flowers at least as delicious.

▶ For 4 people
Easy to prepare   ⊙ 25 min. + 30 min. baking time
330 mL low-fat milk · 50 g honey · 1 tsp dried lavender flowers (also fresh lavender flowers, alternative 7 spices mix) · ½ tsp natural vanilla · lemon zest · 2 eggs · 1 tbsp almond oil

- Combine the milk, honey, lavender, lemon zest, and vanilla, bring the mixture to a boil, and then let it steep for ca. 15 min. Strain through a fine sieve and let it cool.
- Thoroughly mix the eggs with the almond oil and slowly add the milk, stirring continuously. Pour the egg-milk mixture into ovenproof molds and bake covered in a water bath in a preheated 110 °C oven (100 °C convection oven). Small ramekins require ca. 30 min. Then sprinkle unrefined cane sugar on top and caramelize under the broiler with top heat—even better with a Bunsen burner.

Nutritional values per portion
145 calories/ 7 g total fat/ 14 g total carbohydrates/ 6 g protein

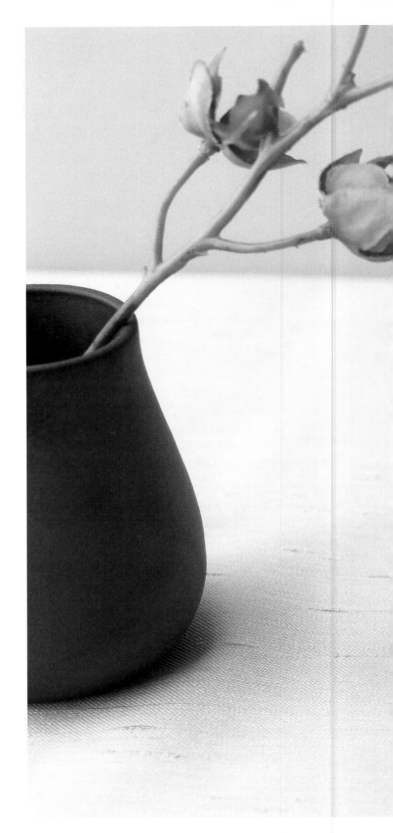

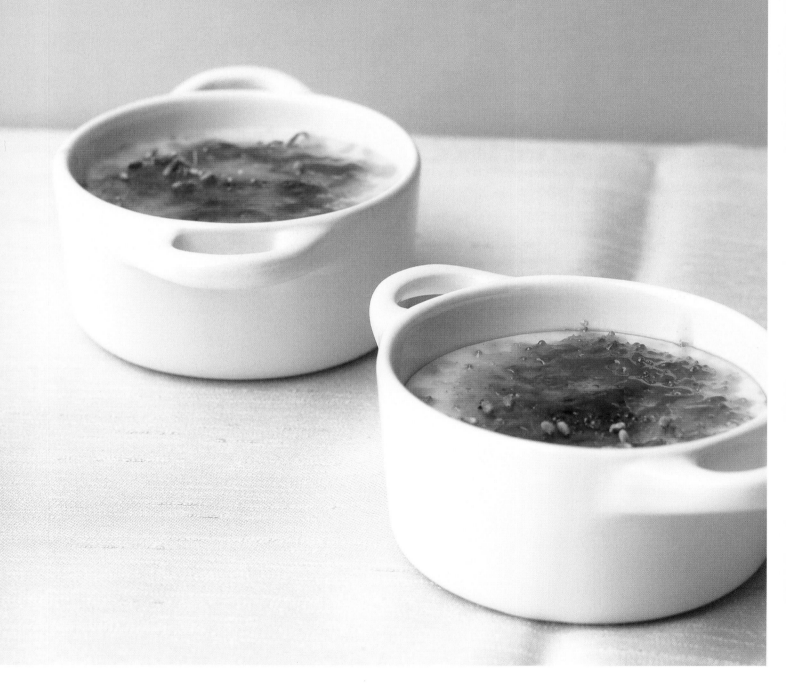

DESSERTS AND CAKES

Quark Dessert

Such a simple recipe, and yet so delicious.

▶ **For 2 people**
Quick to prepare · ⊙ 5 min.
200 g low-fat quark · **1 tbsp** hazelnut oil · **1 tbsp** concentrated fruit juice, honey, or chopped dried fruit · **200 g** fresh fruit · **spices:** vanilla, cinnamon, cocoa, chopped mint, or lemon balm

- Put the quark in a bowl and add the oil and maybe a little water. Mix everything vigorously with a whisk. Whipping the quark with the oil gives it a creamy consistency.
- Add the fruit juice concentrate, honey, or chopped dried fruit—the amount depends on the sweetness of the fruit. Grate or chop the fresh fruit. The finer you process the fruit, the more sweetness it develops. Fold the fruit into the quark. Now add spices or herbs according to taste.

Nutritional values per portion
195 calories / 5 g total fat / 21 g total carbohydrates / 14 g protein

Vanilla Custard with Stewed Apricots

A light custard combined with apricots with a hint of caramel—superb!

▶ **For 2 people**
Easy to prepare · ⊙ 20 min.
250 mL milk · **1 tbsp** unrefined cane sugar · **2 tbsp** pumpkin, finely grated **½ tsp** natural vanilla · **2 tbsp** brown rice, finely ground · **150 g** apricots · **1 tbsp** honey

- Heat the milk. Stir in the sugar, grated pumpkin, vanilla, and ground rice. Stirring continuously, bring the mixture to a boil and simmer for 2 min. Adjust the seasonings and pour into 2 bowls.
- Pit the apricots. Caramelize the honey in a pan and toss very quickly with the apricots. Serve alongside the vanilla custard.

Nutritional values per portion
215 calories / 5 g total fat / 35 g total carbohydrates / 6 g protein

Fennel Strawberry Salad

A dessert with a Sicilian flair, also wonderful as an appetizer.

▶ **For 2 people**
Quick to prepare · ⊙ 10 min.
Juice from 1 lemon · **3 tbsp** canola oil salt/freshly ground pepper · **2 small** fennel bulbs · **100 g** strawberries · **1 tsp** fresh green pepper

- Put the lemon juice, oil, and spices in a bowl and mix. Cut the fennel very finely or grate it, then mix it with the marinade.
- Slice the strawberries into very fine slivers and add carefully to the fennel. Season with the spices and fresh green pepper. Chop the fennel greens and arrange on top.

Nutritional values per portion
180 calories / 15 g total fat / 8 g total carbohydrates / 3 g protein

Sour Cherry and Fig Ice Cream

An ice cream made entirely without conventional sugar.

▶ For 2 people
Good for preparing ahead of time
🕑 20 min. + 2–4 hours freezing time
250 g sour cherries · 50 g dried figs · 100 g bananas · a little cinnamon

▬ Pit the cherries. Finely chop the dried figs and slice the banana. Purée everything together and then freeze the mixture. When frozen, purée with a stick blender or run through a meat grinder. Then fluff it up again with a whisk.

▶ Serving suggestions
Vanilla sauce tastes wonderful with this ice cream.

Nutritional values per portion
175 calories/ 1 g total fat/ 36 g total carbohydrates/ 3 g protein

FACTS

Bratapfel Ice Cream

Just prepare double the recipe and purée and freeze the half that you haven't used. Then purée the whole frozen mixture or run it through the fine attachment in a meat grinder. Fluff the ice cream with a whisk, and you have made sumptuous Bratapfel ice cream. Vanilla sauce is the perfect match for this dish as well.

Bratapfel

A classic winter dish but also marvelous as Bratapfel ice cream.

▶ For 2 people
Budget-friendly
🕑 10 min. + 20 min. baking time
60 g hazelnuts · 1 tsp raisins · 1 tbsp honey · cinnamon · 2 apples · a little lemon juice · 100 mL apple juice

▬ Lightly toast the hazelnuts, let them cool, and grind finely in a food processor. Add the raisins, honey, and a little cinnamon, and depending on the consistency of the honey possibly a little apple juice.
▬ Peel the apples, remove the cores with an apple corer, and fill with the hazelnut mixture. Set the apples in an ovenproof dish, add the apple juice, and bake in a 160 °C oven (145 °C convection oven) for 10–20 min., depending on the variety of apple used.

▶ Serving suggestions
Delicious with vanilla sauce.

Nutritional values per portion
335 calories/ 20 g total fat/ 33 g total carbohydrates/ 5 g protein

Stewed Spiced Pear

Wonderful as a holiday season dessert, especially when combined with the Bratapfel ice cream.

▶ For 2 people
Budget-friendly
🕑 10 min. + 5–10 min. baking time
300 g pears · 1–2 tbsp honey · 1 tbsp hazelnut oil · 50 g sweet cherry juice · natural vanilla · cinnamon · clove · star anise · ginger · 1 large pinch rice flour

▬ Quarter the pears, remove the cores, and cut into wedges. If the peel is very firm, remove that as well.
▬ Brown the honey lightly with the oil in a pan. First add the spices, then the pear wedges. Deglaze with the fruit juice and stew in this until soft. Remove the pear wedges and thicken the liquid a little with the rice flour, then add the pear back in.

▶ Serving suggestions
This is perfect with a vanilla quark crème or even just plain whipped yoghurt.

Nutritional values per portion
180 calories/ 6 g total fat/ 32 g total carbohydrates/ 1 g protein

Strawberry Coconut Balls

The balls also taste delicious as a frozen ice cream confection.

▶ For ca. 500 g
Easy to prepare   ⊙ 25 min.
300 g strawberries · 200 g grated coconut ·
1 tsp honey · a little allspice · a little natural
vanilla

▬ Quarter the strawberries and purée them.
Add the grated coconut, honey, and spices to
the puréed strawberries and mix everything
with a spoon. Let the mixture rest for 15 min.,
form into balls, and refrigerate or freeze.

Nutritional values per recipe
215 calories/ 11 g total fat/ 23 g total
carbohydrates/ 4 g protein

TIP
Remove the balls from the freezer about
15 min. before serving them.

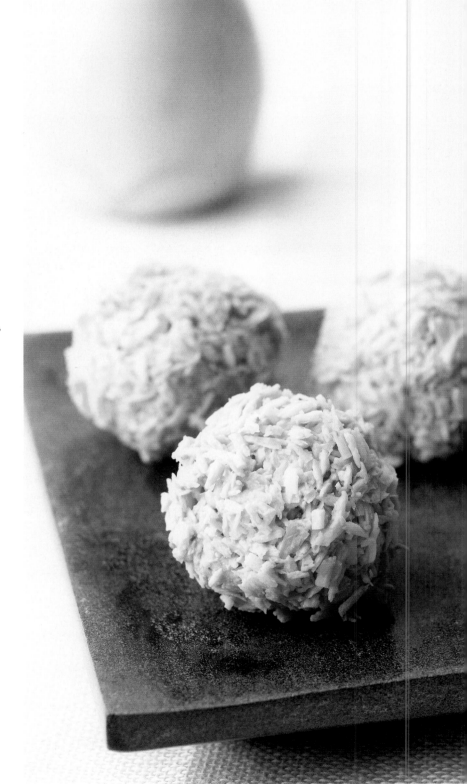

Oat Coconut Confection

Quickly rolled into balls, not too sweet, and just simply good.

▶ For approx. 300 g
Quick to prepare
⊙ 10 min.
80 g heavy cream · 80 g low-fat yoghurt · 80 g wholegrain oatflakes · 80 g grated coconut · 2 tbsp unrefined cane sugar

▬ Whip the cream. Mix all ingredients together. Let everything rest for 15 min. Then form into small balls and roll in grated coconut.

▶ Info
For this recipe, you should use store-bought rolled oats because freshly rolled oats will turn bitter.

▶ Serving suggestions
Serve with a fruit salad.

Nutritional values per recipe
1160 calories/ 84 g total fat/ 80 g total carbohydrates/ 21 g protein

Tip
Store leftover balls in the fridge.

Energy Bars

These bars keep for at least two weeks in a cookie tin.

▶ For 1 baking sheet
Easy to prepare
⊙ 20 min. + 20 min. baking time
For the dough: 200 g wholegrain spelt flour · 75 g butter · 75 g unrefined cane sugar · zest from ½ lemon 60 mL water
For the topping: 200 mL milk · 100 g dried apricots · 100 g hazelnuts

▬ For the dough, finely cube the cold butter, add to the spelt flour, and work it in with two dough scrapers or a pastry blender. Add the remaining ingredients to this mixture and quickly knead everything to form a smooth dough. Roll the dough out thinly and place on a baking sheet. Refrigerate.
▬ For the topping, bring the milk to a boil. Purée the apricots, grind the nuts. Add both to the milk and mix everything. Spread the topping on top of the dough and bake in a 170 °C oven (150 °C convection oven) for 20 min. Then cut into bars and let them cool.

Nutritional values per recipe
2550 calories/ 141 g total fat/ 265 g total carbohydrates/ 54 g protein

Quark Waffles

Not that high in fat but sweet like conventional waffles. Yum!

▶ For 8 waffles
Quick to prepare
⊙ 10 min. + 15 min. baking time
200 g butter · 100 g unrefined cane sugar · 250 g quark · 3 eggs · 300 g wholegrain spelt flour · 1 tsp cream of tartar baking powder · 250 mL milk · lemon zest · natural vanilla

▬ Beat the butter with the unrefined sugar until fluffy. Separate the eggs. Gradually add the egg yolks to the butter-sugar mixture. Whip the quark, add the vanilla and lemon zest, and combine everything with the butter-egg-sugar mixture.
▬ Beat the egg whites until stiff. Mix the flour with the baking powder and stir with the milk into the butter-egg-sugar mixture. Lastly, fold the egg whites gently into the dough and then use a waffle iron to bake the waffles until golden brown.

Nutritional values per waffle
440 calories/ 25 g total fat/ 39 g total carbohydrates/ 13 g protein

Tip
Enjoy the waffles as a sweet main dish with stewed fruit or as a dessert after a main course of soup or salad.

Apple Crumble

Easily prepared and a great substitute for apple pie.

▶ For 1 casserole dish
Good for preparing ahead of time
⏲ 20 min. + 30 min. baking time
50 g hazelnuts · 50 g walnuts · 100 g wholegrain spelt flour · cinnamon · 2 tbsp honey · 2 tbsp hazelnut oil · 3 apples · 1 tbsp raisins

— Finely grind the hazelnuts and walnuts, then mix with the wholegrain flour and a little cinnamon. Stir the honey with the hazelnut oil until well combined. Add to the nut and flour mixture and rub between your fingers to make streusel (crumble).
— Quarter and core the apples and cut into thin slices. Add the raisins, season with a little cinnamon, and mix well. Arrange the apples in a casserole dish, sprinkle the streusel on top, and bake in a 160 °C oven (145 °C convection oven) for 30 min.

▶ Variation
Also delicious with pears, peaches, or apricots. Serve with a fruit sauce or vanilla sauce. Also tastes great with Sour Cherry and Fig Ice Cream (p. 103).

Nutritional values per recipe
1520 calories / 91 g total fat / 146 g total carbohydrates / 30 g protein

Chocolate Cake with Blueberries

A delicious juicy cake!

▶ For 1 cake
Easy to prepare
⏲ 15 min. + 40 min. baking time
3 eggs · 200 g butter · 150 g honey · 350 g wholegrain spelt flour · 1 tsp cream of tartar baking powder · 50 g cocoa powder · 100 mL milk · 100 g blueberries

— Separate the eggs. Beat the egg yolks with the butter (brought to room temperature) and stir in the honey. Beat the egg whites until stiff. Mix the flour with the baking powder and cocoa and stir with the milk into the butter and egg mixture.
— As the last step, gently fold in the stiff egg whites. Pour the dough into a greased baking pan and sprinkle the blueberries on top. Lightly press the berries into the dough. Bake in a 170 °C oven (150 °C convection oven) for ca. 40 min.

▶ Variation
Also tastes wonderful when made with pear wedges or with finely grated quince, which are added to the cocoa and flour mixture.

Nutritional values per cake
3520 calories / 202 g total fat / 347 g total carbohydrates / 80 g protein

Cheesecake à la Buchinger

A quick cheesecake with pear, but without a crust.

▶ For 1 cake
Quick to prepare
⏲ 10 min. + 30 min. baking time
500 g quark (low-fat) · 40 g hazelnut butter · 100 g wildflower honey · 2 eggs · natural vanilla · grated zest from 1 untreated orange and 1 untreated lemon · 400 g pears

— Mix the quark with the hazelnut butter and the honey. Separate the eggs. Stir the egg yolks with the vanilla and lemon and orange zest into this mixture. Quarter the pears, remove the cores, and cut into wedges. If the peel is very firm, remove that as well.
— Arrange the pears on the bottom of a springform pan lined with parchment paper (26 cm in diameter). Beat the egg whites until stiff and fold carefully into the quark mixture. Spread this on top of the pear wedges. Bake the cake for ca. 30 min. in a 160 °C oven (145 °C convection oven).

▶ Variation
This cake also works well with blueberries or sour cherries.

Nutritional values per cake
1310 calories / 40 g total fat / 146 g total carbohydrates / 91 g protein

▶ Cheesecake à la Buchinger

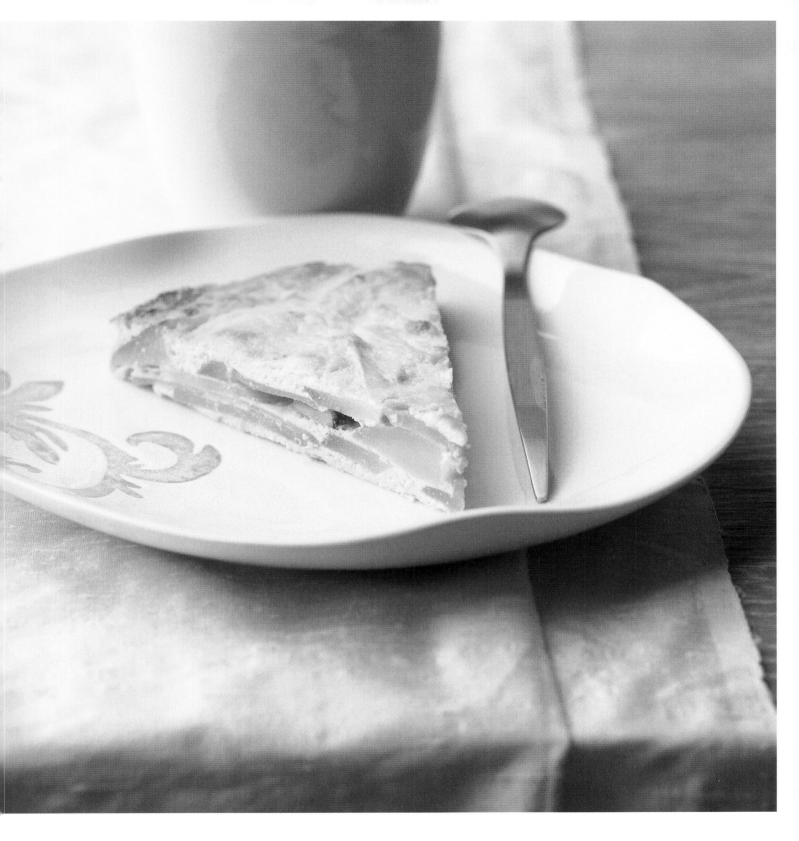

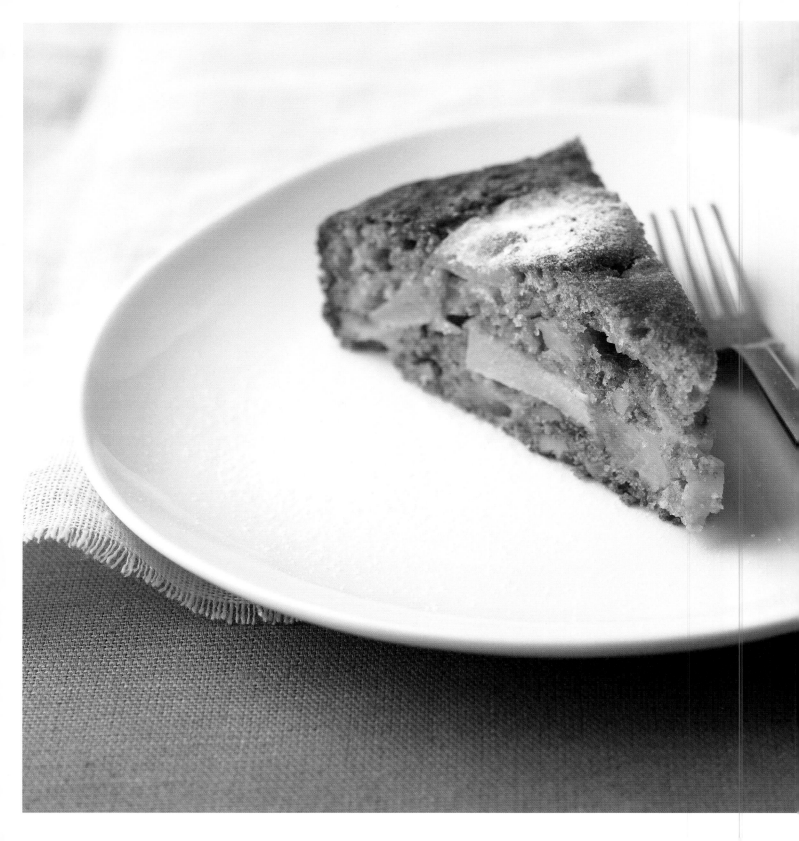

Quince Cake

With natural sweetness from apple juice concentrate.

- Take the butter, eggs, and apple juice concentrate out of the fridge for a few hours before baking to bring them up to room temperature. Peel and core the quinces. Heat the peels and cores in a pot with 250 mL water and simmer covered for 15 min.
- Cut the quinces into 1-cm cubes. Strain the quince cooking liquid, add the unrefined sugar, and simmer the quince cubes in this liquid for 30 min. Then drain the quince cubes over a sieve. Save the liquid (you can use it as quince syrup).
- Separate the eggs. Beat the egg whites until stiff and refrigerate. Whip the butter. Add the egg yolks to the butter one at a time and continue beating until they are completely incorporated into the batter. Continue whipping the batter and slowly add the apple juice concentrate—give the batter time to absorb it. Mix the flour with the baking powder, spices, and salt.
- Add the flour mixture, walnuts, drained quince cubes, and lemon zest to the batter and fold everything in carefully. Lastly fold the egg whites gently into the mixture. Pour the dough into a greased springform pan and bake in a 160 °C oven (preferably convection oven, otherwise 175 °C top and bottom heat) for 50 min. After half the baking time, cover with parchment paper or aluminum foil—if necessary—to prevent the cake from getting too brown.

Nutritional values per cake
5740 calories/ 370 g total fat/ 488 g total carbohydrates/ 103 g protein

TIP

If the butter and egg yolk mixture cannot absorb the apple juice concentrate completely, continue beating while you sit the bowl in a lukewarm water bath (ca. 37 °C), until any flakes that might have formed are dissolved.

▶ For 1 cake
Requires a little more time
⊘ 25 min. + 1½ hours cooking and baking time

250 g butter
5 eggs
300 mL apple juice concentrate
350 g quinces
250 mL water
50 g unrefined cane sugar
250 g wholegrain spelt flour
2 tsp cream of tartar baking powder
Cinnamon
Natural vanilla
Zest from 1 untreated lemon
Pinch salt
160 g walnuts

109

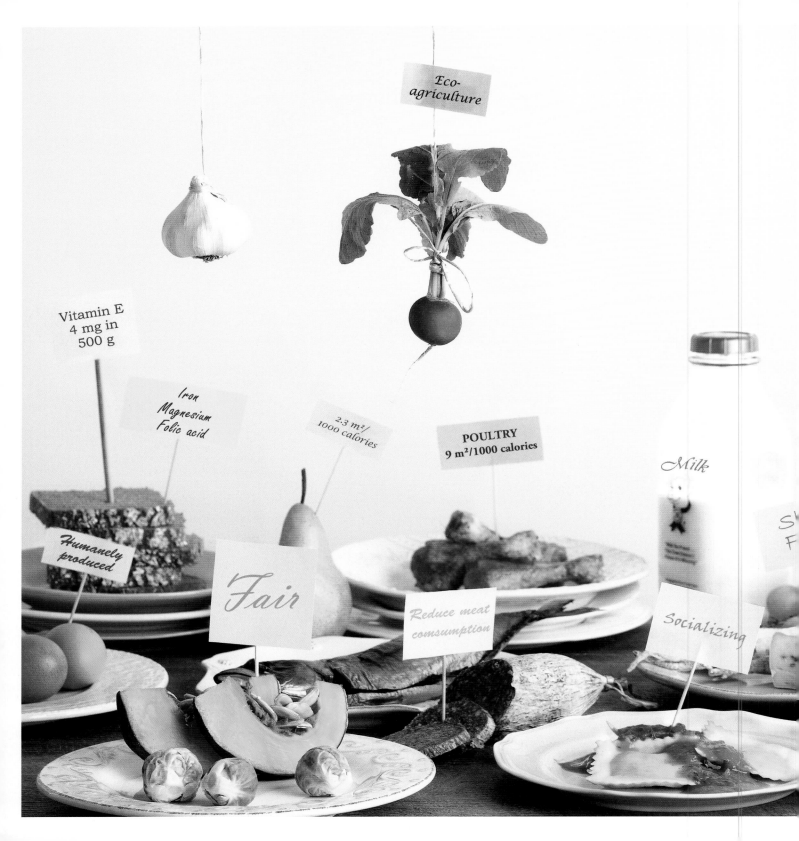

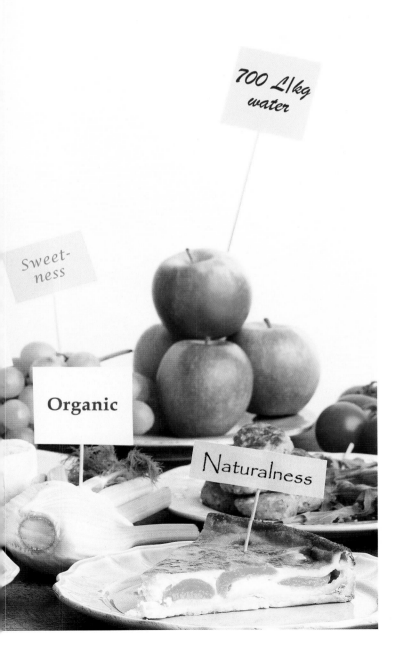

Sustainable Eating: The Basics

How do cow pastures help us secure global food supplies? How much "virtual water" is contained in, for example, 1 kg (or 1 lb) of potatoes? Which organic farming associations have renounced the use of animal feed from developing countries? What are the arguments for local and seasonal products? What are natural foods? Why is Fair Trade fair?

More Plant Products—and Fewer Animal Products

In most industrial countries, much more animal products are consumed today than just 50 years ago. The latest figures for average world meat consumption indicate consumption of approximately 47 kg (103 lb) per person per year, approximately 900 g (2 lb) per week.[10] The recommended amount per person per week, however, is considerably lower: approximately 300 g (0.7 lb) of meat—as well 150 g (0.3 lb) of fish and up to two eggs.[2,9] The following chapter will explain why a primarily plant-based diet is not only good for our health but also has ecological, social, and economic advantages.

Environmental Stresses from Agriculture and Livestock Farming

According to International Energy Agency (IEA) estimates for 2009, greenhouse gas emissions for the average person in the United States or European Union were 17 or 7 tons per year respectively.[11] The sustainable amount for the climate, however, is currently estimated at only 2 tons per person per year.[12] We citizens of rich industrialized countries therefore have to drastically reduce our greenhouse gas emissions by up to 80–90% if we want to reach the goal of sustainability.

Whereas agriculture is responsible for 14% of all greenhouse gas (GHG) emissions produced worldwide, approximately 18% of all GHG emissions can be attributed to the production of animal-based foods.[13] The manufacture of these foods generates several times the amount of greenhouse gases than plant-based foods. To cultivate crops for animal fodder, a lot of energy is necessary, especially in the chemical industry, in order to produce mineral nitrogen fertilizer for conventional agriculture. The conversion of plant products into animal products, moreover, is often quite inefficient. As a result, their greenhouse gas balance sheet declines sharply. To this, we further have to add those greenhouse gases that are produced during rearing, keeping, processing and so on, either from energy use or by the animals themselves, such as methane and nitrous oxide in their excretions (see Facts p. 113).[13]

As a rule, plant-based foods also require considerably less water for their production than animal-based ones. What we refer to as "virtual water" is not the water that the product actually contains but the "invisible" water that was used for its production and processing. The production of 1 kg of beef in intensive livestock operations, for example, requires more than 15 000 L of water. Most notably, this includes irrigation for the cultivation of feed. The production of 1 kg of potatoes, by contrast, requires only 287 L of water (see table).[14,15]

Virtual water content of plant- and animal-based foods[14, 15]

Animal-based Foods		Plant-based Foods	
	Virtual water (L/kg food)		Virtual water (L/kg food)
Beef	15 415	Wheat	1 827
Cheese	3 178	Bananas	790
Pork	5 988	Apples	822
Poultry	4 325	Potatoes	287
Eggs	3 266	Tomatoes	214

The "import of virtual water" is highly problematic when agricultural products come from countries that suffer from water shortages but use large amounts of water for irrigation. Take for example strawberries imported from Israel, which are grown in the desert with elaborate irrigation systems, or early potatoes from Morocco or Egypt. In ecological terms, this makes no sense since you can certainly store domestic potatoes through the spring.

How Cow Pastures Can Help Secure Global Food Supplies

The production of animal-based foods requires much more agricultural land than the production of plant-based foods. In order to produce 1000 kcal in the form of beef (corresponding to approx. 900 g or 2 lb), we need more than 30 m² of productive land. This includes areas for pasturing as well as for the cultivation of additional feedstuffs. For 1000 kcal in the form of vegetables (corresponding to approx. 3 kg or 6.6 lb), on the other hand, an average area of only 1.7 m² is required (see table on p. 114).[16]

Approximately one-third of globally available arable land is used for the cultivation of animal feed.[17] If these fields were used for growing crops like grain, potatoes, or legumes instead, which could be utilized directly to feed humans, considerably more food would be available to secure global food supplies. The use of fields

FACTS

From the Climate Perspective, Are Cows a Problem?

Ruminants (e.g., cows, sheep, goats) produce the very harmful greenhouse gas methane during digestion. Does this mean that cows are in the doghouse from the climate perspective?

Why Pasturing Is Better for the Climate

When it comes to ruminants we must differentiate clearly between the different husbandry systems. The reason for this is that permanent grassland that is not tilled into cultivated fields for years at a time has the potential to absorb carbon dioxide (CO_2) from the atmosphere. Grass plants use photosynthesis to store large amounts of carbon in their deep, widely branching roots—for the entire length of the year. When the roots die off, earthworms and so on transform them into fertile humus, which constitutes a significant climate-friendly carbon reservoir.

Note: The climate benefit of cows on sustainably managed permanent pasture does not apply, however, to high-performance cows in intensive livestock operations. These graze little or not at all, but eat protein- and energy-rich feed concentrates that are often imported. Soy, which is an important ingredient in feed concentrates, is often produced in countries like Brazil or Paraguay on fields that have been converted from tropical rainforest to agricultural land. This process emits large amounts of greenhouse gases. In addition, the rainforest is then no longer available for sequestering CO_2, which gives cause for serious concern from a climate standpoint, among other things. The production of feed concentrates, moreover, requires large amounts of energy: the energy-intensive synthetic nitrogen fertilizers used for this purpose constitute an important contribution to greenhouse gases. In organic agriculture these are replaced with so-called green manures with grass and clover seeds, to improve the fertility of the soil. The harvested green fodder also serves as a good source of additional protein for ruminants.

Cows, Sheep, and Goats Are Not Climate Killers Per Se

All in all, the formation of humus means that sustainable pasturing of ruminants on permanent grassland has considerable benefits for the climate compared to conventional methods. This fact is sharply at odds with their widespread image as climate killers. From the climate perspective, a certain—but clearly reduced—amount of milk (including cheese and other dairy products) and meat from ruminants is therefore by all means acceptable—as long as it comes from animals on permanent pasture.[18]

Land requirements for animal- and plant-based foods (m² cultivated land per edible food energy)[16]

Animal-based Foods		Plant-based Foods	
	Land requirement (m²/1000 kcal)		Land requirement (m²/1000 kcal)
Beef	31.2 (5.3 + 25.9*)	Oleiferous fruits	3.2
Poultry	9.0	Fruit	2.3
Pork	7.3	Legumes	2.2
Eggs	6.0	Vegetables	1.7
Whole milk	5.0 (1.2 + 3.8*)	Grains	1.1

* Pastureland

FACTS

Speaking of Land Competition

In developing countries, the cultivation of export products has caused land competition for food production for the local population. Besides animal feeds like cassava, soy, and corn, this also includes tropical fruits, coffee, tea, cocoa, tobacco, cotton, and flowers. In African countries, for example, export production covers approx. 5–20% of the total area in agricultural production. The remaining land would be sufficient to supply the African population with food. But a conflict exists in qualitative terms: the best soil and most labor are often used for the production of export goods. Many governments additionally promote export-oriented farming with credit programs and by providing seeds and fertilizer. Because export products can generally fetch higher profits, this can lead to the neglect of food production for personal consumption and local markets.

---

for the production of animal feed over food supplies in developing countries can lead to competition over arable land and thereby contribute to world hunger (see Facts). Importing animal feed from developing countries is consequently a highly problematic practice.

In addition, the production of animal-based foods creates so-called refinement losses since the animals consume a large part of the energy from their feed for their own metabolism. Depending on the species, feeding methods, and so on, they convert only about a third or less into meat, milk, or eggs. Thus farmers must feed many times the calories from plant-based feed to produce a single calorie of animal-based food.[4]

This picture changes, however, when ruminants primarily eat grass on pasture. By pasturing cattle, sheep, and goats, farmers are able to utilize existing permanent grassland for the production of high-quality foods. In most cases, existing pastureland is otherwise not usable for food production for humans. This is because when topsoil is thin, the risk of erosion from wind or water makes ploughing and the conversion into cultivated fields a questionable choice. The same applies to steep locations in low mountain ranges, the Alpine Foothills, the Alps, or wet areas near the coast. The conversion into cultivated fields, moreover, would release large amounts of CO_2, which is highly undesirable in terms of climate protection. From this perspective, we can even speak of a "refinement gain" when pastureland is utilized by ruminants. When grazed on permanent pasture, cows and other ruminants are not food competitors for humans because they do not—unlike pigs and poultry—depend on feed from cultivated land like grains and soy. If we look at the land used worldwide for agricultural production, by far the largest percentage is actually in permanent pasture (69%). The rest is annual crops (29%) and permanent crops like orchards and vineyards (2%).[19] The production of milk and meat from ruminants in extensive and sustainable livestock operations on perennial pastureland therefore does indeed make sense. When feed concentrates are avoided, it is an important contribution to world food supplies, especially for developing countries.[18]

Animal husbandry is, moreover, an important source of income for farmers. More than 800 million people worldwide depend on grasslands for their livelihood.[20] Ruminants on permanent pasture also help preserve the local diversity of our cultural landscape, because pastures would otherwise become overgrown with bush or forest—for our leisure and for tourism a priceless asset.

Reducing Meat Consumption: A Healthier Diet

When we eat less animal-based and instead more plant-based foods we generally also consume less harmful fats and instead more complex long-chain carbohydrates. These also contain more dietary fiber. Complex carbohydrates promote lower blood sugar levels, as long as the food has not been too highly processed and the dietary fiber has not been removed. In most cases, plant-based foods—notably plant oils, nuts, and oilseeds (e.g., sunflower, pumpkin, flax, and sesame seeds)—boast a healthier composition of fatty acids than animal-based foods (such as meat and sausage). The latter, on the other hand, tend to contain considerable amounts of potentially harmful ingredients like saturated fatty acids, cholesterol, purine, and salt.

Plant-based foods like whole grains, legumes, vegetables, and fruits by contrast are characterized by a high nutrient density. This means that they contain an abundance of vital ingredients like vitamins and minerals (when measured against their dietary energy). Healthy dietary fiber and phytochemicals (e.g., phytosterols or carotenoids) are found almost exclusively in products made from plants. Generally speaking, plant-based foods at the same time supply less energy and we tend to feel sated after consuming even a small amount of energy. However, when we eat a lot of meat, sausage, and eggs, we run the risk of ingesting more calories than necessary.

For these reasons, a primarily plant-based diet with lots of vegetables, fruits, legumes, and whole grains is helpful in the prevention of various diet-related disorders, for example, excess weight, type 2 diabetes, cancer, cardiovascular disorders, and high blood pressure.[8,21]

Humane Livestock Farming Has Its Price

When buying meat and sausage as well as dairy products and eggs it is important to look for high quality. Animal products should not be cheap mass-produced goods, even if many refrigerated displays suggest the opposite. Meat, sausage, eggs, and milk from animals that were raised and fed humanely and organically have their price so that farmers can earn fair wages for their complex labor. When we choose to eat meat and meat products less frequently we can indulge in the best quality and still save money.

How Good Is Organic Food—
For Us, For Others, and For Nature?

The increasing intensification of agriculture is contributing to a number of different environmental problems. Soil and water can, for example, become polluted by nitrogen, phosphates, and pesticides. The bill arrives directly on our dinner plate and in the cup—potentially harmful residues in our food and drinking water.

What many people do not know is that agriculture is responsible for a considerable portion of greenhouse gas emissions. Other possible effects are soil compaction, soil erosion, and decline in biological diversity. When we stress soils, plants, animals, and raw materials beyond their limits there are local and global consequences. One way out of this dilemma is offered by sustainable or ecological/organic agriculture (these terms have the same meaning). Organic agriculture is also good for our health and can offer economic and social benefits.

Organic: Better for the Environment

For a number of environmental reasons, food from ecological agriculture is more acceptable than products from conventional production. Ecological crop cultivation, for example, requires less energy: based on 1 ha and depending on the crop type, roughly 30% to half the energy is used, leading to a corresponding reduction in greenhouse gas emissions.[22] But

yields are also usually lower in organic cultivation. One study has shown great variability in both forms of agriculture when the balance sheet of greenhouse gas emissions was correlated with equal yields: sometimes it was the ecological, sometimes the conventional operation that turned out to be more favorable for the climate. When averaging out all the farms in the study though, the organic producers came out roughly a quarter more favorable, in spite of lower yields. This is because, among other factors, they forego the use of mineral nitrogen fertilizer, which requires a large amount of energy to manufacture. Ecological cultivation, moreover, facilitates a greater build-up of humus, which absorbs CO_2 from the atmosphere (see p. 113).[23]

One particularly relevant problem in agriculture is the emission of nitrous oxide (N_2O), which is 300 times more harmful to the climate than CO_2. It is formed during the breakdown of mineral fertilizer in conventional production and of manure (i.e., from

animal waste) in both organic and conventional agriculture.

In livestock management, the effects on the climate depend on many factors, most notably feed quality, lifetime production of the animals, and manure management. Energy consumption is lower in ecological livestock operations. When organic farms take advantage of all opportunities for optimization they can be less harmful to the climate than conventional operations.[24, 25] One advantage of organic agriculture is the extensive use of feed straight from the producer's own farm. When animal feed is produced right there on the spot it provides the greatest possible transparency, and transport over large distances is eliminated. The ideal is a closed agricultural loop in which plants, animals, and soils are all interconnected. When feed for the animal comes directly from the farm, it strengthens the natural cycles.

Organic agriculture supports natural soil fertility and thereby increases humus content and lowers the tendency to erosion. The degradation and erosion of soil due to conventional agricultural practices among other factors is a significant environmental problem—worldwide, billions of tons of fertile topsoil are lost each year.[26]

In comparison with conventional agriculture, we tend to find more naturalized areas in organic agriculture (e.g., wetlands, mixed orchards with meadows, field margins). Ecologically cultivated areas therefore provide more habitats for animals and plants and thus promote biological diversity. As a result, pests cannot spread as quickly and fruit blossoms are pollinated naturally.[27]

In addition, organic agriculture foregoes genetic engineering. On the whole, ecological agriculture combines productivity with the avoidance of environmental stresses and the preservation of natural resources.

Why don't you visit an organic farmer near you? For example, find a farm at www.localharvest.org, www.local-farmers-markets.co.uk, or www.localfoods.org.uk.

Organic Foods Are Healthier

Many studies have shown that organic foods on the one hand contain markedly less residues of nitrates, pesticides, and veterinary drugs. The main reason for this is that the use of synthetic fertilizers, pesticides, and veterinary drugs in organic farming and animal husbandry is either prohibited or limited to a degree dependent on individual national standards.

On the other hand, foods like tuber and root vegetables (e.g., carrots, beets) from organic production contain larger amounts of principal nutrients than conventional products (related to their lower water content). With regard to vitamins and minerals, the differences between ecologically and conventionally produced fruits and vegetables are hardly noticeable—only the vitamin C content tends to be higher. In addition, organic fruits and vegetables often contain more phytochemicals, which among other benefits have antioxidant, antibacterial, or immune-strengthening effects and contribute to the prevention of cardiovascular disorders and cancer.[28]

Many people buy organically grown vegetables and fruits as well as animal products because they taste better. Organic carrots, for example, often have a more intense flavor than conventional ones. Moreover, we can often find a greater range of varieties, for example, in the case of apples, tomatoes, and potatoes.

In the organic sector, food is generally processed more gently. Irradiation of food to increase its shelf life is, for example, rejected, and the range of permitted additives such as colorants and preservatives is much more limited. As a rule, not even natural or nature-identical aromas are added.

Organic Agriculture Secures Livelihoods and Creates Jobs

As a rule, the higher profits in organic farming offer farmers greater security in their livelihoods, but it does require more labor. In the last few years, however, the downward pressure on prices has also had a negative effect on producer prices in the organic sector—and therefore also on their income levels. Nevertheless, additional jobs are created due to the high labor

---

TIP

Food Boxes Delivered Directly to Your Home

Many organic farmers deliver "food boxes" directly to your home. In most cases you can choose between a subscription (a variety of seasonal fruits and vegetables) and individually assembled food boxes. You can often also order bread, dairy products, and meat at the same time, by phone or fax and also through the internet. In rural areas, with no health food store nearby, farm stores on organic farms offer yet another option.

requirements, on-site processing, and direct marketing through farm stores and farmers' markets.

Social Aspects of Organic Agriculture

Some organic agriculture associations consciously discourage the use of imported animal feeds from developing countries (see table). One reason for this is that the land for the production of such feed for export stands in direct competition for land with the local population.

A survey of organic farmers showed that they were happier in their work after the conversion from conventional to organic agriculture.[29] Organic farming often also implies additional social and cultural benefits, such as kindergarten and school farms, farms for therapy and for integrating people with disabilities or mental illness, as well as farms that include older people in the operation.

There are different labels by which you can recognize organically produced food. These reflect various quality levels and can be bought in different stores (see p. 133).

In most cases, organic and Fair Trade associations discourage animal feeds from developing countries (personal survey of selected associations, 2012)

Association	Is Animal Feed Imported from Developing Countries?
Demeter	Animals must be fed with biodynamic or organic fodder; no conventional fodder or genetically modified (GM) feed is allowed (with the exception of minerals). Each national member state is free to set higher standards than the Demeter International (DI) standard. In most cases, regional fodder is used, although DI standards permit organic fodder from outside the farm or cooperative, including from abroad—but not from developing countries.
Go Organic/ Soil Association	Campaigns actively against the use of genetic modification technologies, as the vast majority of grain imported into the EU for livestock feed is of genetic manipulation origin, specifically grown for the purpose of being exported as animal fodder. This organization also underlines the importance of not relying so heavily on imports, including the importation of grain for livestock feed, with reference to the issue of local food security.
World Fair Trade Organization	Recognizes the importance of addressing this issue both on local and international levels in relation to food security and food sovereignty in developing countries. Activities entail member involvement in discussions, national forums, and campaigns.
Sustainable Agriculture Network and Rainforest Alliance	As part of this organization's Standard for Sustainable Cattle Production Systems, farms must produce most of their own feed and fodder, except when impossible due to atypical adverse conditions. In addition, selection of forage species should include the consideration of agro-ecological conditions, production rates, nutritional value, and resistance to pests or adverse climatic conditions.
EU Regulation 2092/91 (Organic) vs. US organic regulations for livestock	US organic regulations require 100% organic feed (except for approved feed additives and approved synthetic inert ingredients and milk replacer in case of an emergency). EU Regulation 2092/91 previously allowed feed from conventional sources, including 5% for herbivores, and up to 15% for other species until 2007, with a decreasing share until 2011. From 2012 onwards, however, EU organic regulations also require 100% organic feed. EU regulations specify feed formula per species whereas US organic regulations do not. Importantly, EU organic regulations require that for herbivores at least 50% of the feed must come from the farm unit itself or a cooperating farm, whereas US organic regulations do not include this stipulation.

Labels for Organic Foods

As a customer who buys organic products maybe you have also heard something like this before: "Organic simply contains the same stuff, you just pay more for it" or "But there is cheating going on everywhere anyway." Nevertheless, organic certification has been legally regulated and controlled since 1990 (Organic Foods Production Act) in the United States and since 1991 in the European Union (see new EU Eco-Logo below). Packaging now displays a number of organic labels, seals, or certifications.

Trademarks of Organic Farming Associations

Many organic products also carry the logos of international, national, regional, or local organic farming or certification associations. With these symbols you can trust that the product satisfies even stricter quality guidelines than those required by EU or USDA regulations. Members of these organizations include both large and small organic producers and organic processing plants. Individual commercial producers may also distribute products carrying an organic label, which must adhere to EU or USDA law regulating organic products and processing.

The USDA Organic Seal (Organic Certification Logo)

The United States Department of Agriculture (USDA) organic seal was introduced in 1990 as a national, standardized seal of certification, and verifies that raw or processed agricultural and livestock products are produced according to USDA organic regulations. For more details, including a definition of USDA organic standards, go to the webpage of the National Organic Program: www.ams.usda.gov/nop.

The New EU Eco-Logo

This certification has been in existence since 1991 and is legally mandatory for all organic products. There is a new logo since 2010. More information at www.ec.europa.eu/agriculture/organic/home_en.

www.ec.europa.eu/
agriculture/organic

www.usda.gov

www.seedalliance.
org

www.tilth.org

www.qai-inc.com

www.ccof.org

www.demeter.net

www.demeter-
usa.org

www.soilassociation.
org

www.organicfarmers.
org.uk

www.mofga.org

www.cog.ca

www.organic-
biologique.ca

www.nasaa.com.au

Regional and Seasonal—Your Best Choice

The shorter the distance that a food travels to our plates the fresher and higher in vitamins it can be. This sounds logical. Why is it then that exports have increased in the last few decades? One reason: so-called low-wage countries produce much more cheaply than our local farmers could ever do. For this reason products like Chinese onions end up on Western supermarket shelves.

Our food is sometimes transported halfway around the globe before we buy it. Transport within a country is also a factor, such as deliveries of fruit, grain, or milk from distant states or areas to another—even though these products are also being produced locally. Food also travels far distances for specific intermediate steps during processing. North Sea shrimp, for example, are transported by refrigerated truck to Morocco for peeling—and then back into the shrimp sandwich on the North Sea island of Sylt.

Each season features special foods whose arrival we have anticipated for months. Think here of the many kinds of berries in summer—a pleasure worth waiting for. To buy fresh fruit and vegetables from the area makes sense only when they are seasonal as well, that is, when they are able to grow in open fields instead of in energy-intensive heated greenhouses. When you shop according to which foods are in season, you can buy the best regional fruits and vegetables from open fields. And by doing so, you do the climate and your own health a favor at the same time. In addition, we can hereby support our neighborhood farmers.

Food Transport Wastes Energy and Stresses the Environment

Food transport is indispensable but it burdens the climate. We *can* make a difference, however: the amount of greenhouse gas emissions depends on the distance travelled and on the means of transport. Shorter transport routes can reduce our carbon footprint. In this context, efficient marketing structures are important because inefficiently used means of transport as well as those with limited loading space are harmful to the climate.

The most common method of transport for food is by truck, which carries a relatively high carbon load. In contrast, the same transport by train produces only a third as many greenhouse gases. Extremely detrimental to the environment is transport by air, which causes the highest greenhouse gas emissions.[30] Air transport is used primarily for some highly perishable foods—like certain vegetables and fruits, and certain seafood and meat.[7,31] In this context, less is very obviously more, because reduced freight volumes are not only beneficial for the climate but also mean less noise and less use of land for road construction.

Does food really need to be grown under cover? This is problematic because heated greenhouses and plastic tunnels require very large amounts of energy in winter, mostly heating oil or natural gas. Growing vegetables and fruits in their proper season in open fields is much more beneficial to the climate than production out of season.

Supporting Small and Medium-sized Operations

When we buy products that are locally produced and processed, we support smaller and medium-sized operations and thereby preserve local jobs. Regional cooperation between farmers, processors, retailers, and consumers helps secure livelihoods and strengthens the local economy. In many cases, farmers have teamed up in producer associations that market jointly. In the United States you can find out more about farmers' markets through, for example, www.local-harvest.org/farmers-markets, and in the United Kingdom, for example, under www.local-farmers-markets.co.uk and www.localfoods.org.uk.

Regional Structures Build Trust

Easily manageable regional structures create transparency and build trust for all involved parties. Let's give illegal practices and food scandals the boot! Locally and seasonally produced foods also contribute to a sustainable eating culture and take us back to our roots. Regional specialties and biological diversity are once again highly esteemed in gourmet gastronomy. Many top chefs have returned to working with old, almost forgotten local vegetable varieties, such as the Bodega Red potato or Boston Marrow squash. It is precisely because sweet juicy cherries and asparagus are not available all year long and their season is relatively short that we look forward to them with such anticipation. And lastly, by following the natural fluctuations of seasonal offerings, we automatically build variety into our diet.

TIP

"You Have to Eat What You Want to Rescue"

The Slow Food organization is a movement that is concerned with, among other issues, biodiversity. They created the motto above. The project "Ark of Taste" lists more than 1000 locally used animal and plant species worldwide that have been forgotten or gone out of fashion, for example because potatoes are too small or the livestock puts weight on too slowly. Moreover, vegetable varieties like Sibley squash or Orange Oxheart tomato are all open-pollinated and not hybrids. Hybrids have been developed by the seed companies: they do not grow seeds for next year's sowing and thus force the farmers to buy new seed every year. If you want to ensure the continued existence of this diversity, you should include these products on your menu to support their sale. Maybe you will also find food in your area that you can buy to support the preservation of a species? For the United States it is worth taking a look at the webpage www.slowfoodusa.org. Whether New Hampshire chicken, Narragansett turkey, or American Plains bison, all of these are almost forgotten regional specialties.

Local Fruits and Vegetables Are Usually Fully Ripened

Many people just don't know how good fresh tomatoes taste straight from the garden. Fruits and vegetables that come from far away are often harvested unripe for the long transport. Local products, however, have more time; they are allowed to ripen fully in the field before the harvest. We can taste and smell the difference. In addition, they have yet another essential benefit that we sometimes may not be able to detect with our senses but that our body appreciates: they are higher in essential and healthy ingredients such as different vitamins and phytochemicals (including aromas, which cause the more intense flavor of local products). Ripened open-air vegetables, moreover, generally contain fewer harmful residues than greenhouse goods, for example, nitrates and pesticides.[2]

Local foods can often be recognized by specific logos. The following examples of logos are all from regional food hubs across the United States. Food hubs are defined as businesses or organizations that actively manage the aggregation, distribution, and marketing of food products that come from local and regional producers. These logos can serve as shopping guides even if the certification standards for some of them could still use some improvement. The second group of logos represents the best combination of all—organic foods that are locally produced.

Tip

If you are not sure exactly about the specific harvest times for vegetables and fruits, a glance at a seasonal calendar might help. This can easily be accessed by searching for "seasonal food" in the internet!

Logos for Regional Products (US Examples)

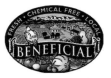

www.beneficialfarm.
com

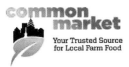

www.commonmarket-
phila.org

www.farmfresh.org

www.gorgegrown.com

www.greenbeandelivery.
com

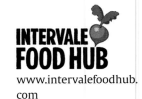

www.intervalefoodhub.
com

www.redtomato.org

www.tusimbolo.org

Logos for Regional Organic Foods (US Examples)

www.albafarmers.org

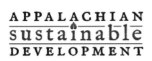

www.asdevelio.org

www.cooppartners.coop

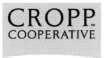

www.farmers.coop

www.viacampesina.org/en

Natural Is the Order of the Day—Especially in Our Diet

Who hasn't heard this: "I'll just pick something up from the Vietnamese place." "I'll quickly heat something up for us"? In this way, we often quell our hunger in between meals and on the side, while we continue working, surfing the internet, or watching TV.

Our accelerated personal and work lives cause us more and more often to fall back on heavily processed foods and ready-made meals, as well as snacks and sweets. These products tend to contain a lot of fat, sugar, salt, and dietary energy, but at the same time contain less essential and health-promoting ingredients per calorie; they are thus marked by low nutrient density. Quite often they include colorants and preservatives, aromas, or other additives, which our body and sense organs don't need.

Industrial processing as well as transport and packaging, moreover, consume energy, resulting in the emission of greenhouse gases and pollutants. Even water is used in large amounts for food processing.

As we cook with lots of ready-made foods, the knowledge around the agricultural product and the cooking-related experiences are increasingly lost, but how much pleasure and enjoyment are we giving up? Cooking is, after all, a wonderful opportunity for relaxing and slowing down. Especially when we cook for good friends (or with them), choose our ingredients with care, and prepare them with love, we can clearly see how creative, sensual, and meaningful cooking is.

Foods as Natural as Possible

When we keep foods as close to their natural state as possible they generally contain more essential and health-promoting ingredients than processed products. The reason for this is that vitamins, minerals, dietary fiber, and phytochemicals are often reduced or removed during processing. Less processed foods additionally tend to contain less fat, sugar, and salt.

Grain serves as a good example to demonstrate this nutrient loss. During the industrial manufacturing of white flour the nutrient-rich surface layers and germ bud of the whole grain are for the most part removed. In whole-grain flour, however, the whole kernel is ground, and the nutrients in it are almost completely preserved (see table, p. 138)

The maxim "as natural as possible" does not mean, however, that we should eat everything unprocessed or raw. Rather, we strive for a healthy mixture of heated and unheated foods: as a rule of thumb, roughly half of each. Depending on your tolerance and preference you can also eat one-third to two-thirds unheated. Certain processing methods do, however, also increase desirable ingredients, as, for example, by sprouting seeds or with lactic acid fermentation (e.g., sauerkraut and sour milk products). These processing methods even increase wholesomeness.

And when you buy basic staples in their pure form—that is, minimally processed or not at all—you also avoid food additives like preservatives, dyes, and aromas.

More Processing, More Greenhouse Gases

The calculation is logical indeed: substances that have been processed more heavily have also consumed more energy and thereby caused more greenhouse gases. Greenhouse gas emissions for the production of dried fruits like apple rings, for example, are 40 times higher than for fresh apples. By drinking water (with the

123

Selected ingredients in 500 g wholewheat bread and white bread[32]

Ingredient	Important for	Wholewheat Bread		White Bread	
Vitamin B$_1$	Strong nerves	1.15 mg	100%	0.45 mg	39%
Vitamin E	Good defense	4 mg	100%	3 mg	75%
Folic acid	Vital cells	125 µg	100%	75 µg	60%
Magnesium	Active muscles	300 mg	100%	120 mg	40%
Iron	Healthy blood	10 mg	100%	3.5 mg	35%
Dietary fiber	Active intestine	42 g	100%	15 g	36%

Percentages refer to the maximum possible amount of the ingredient in bread
(wholewheat bread = maximum = 100%).

exception of bottled mineral water that has come long distances) instead of sodas we can save 85% of the resource consumption and harmful emissions because the manufacture of sugar in particular is extremely energy-intensive. By choosing diluted apple juice over soda, the environmental impact drops by half. Manufacturing beer produces 90 times more greenhouse gases than mineral water.[33]

Cooling (and freezing) and heating also produce considerable amounts of greenhouse gases. Frozen French fries thus produce 29 times more greenhouse gases than fresh potatoes.[34] Sparingly processed foods not only help save energy, water, and greenhouse gases, they can help us avoid many kilometers of transport between the individual processing steps taken in other foods. In addition, transport packaging is almost eliminated.

Our Wallets Are Happy

Sparingly processed or completely unprocessed staples tend to be cheaper because cost-intensive processing steps are eliminated. There are, however, some exceptions such as heavily processed refined flour, which is cheaper than unmilled whole grain. As a general rule, though, ready-made products, sweets, and alcoholic beverages come with disproportionately high prices—especially when measured against their low health value. By purchasing less heavily processed foods, we additionally support smaller and medium-sized cottage industries. This secures livelihoods and preserves or creates local jobs.

Eating Is a Social Event

If you want to give your family, friends, or colleagues a culinary surprise, chances are you won't serve them a ready-made meal. The anticipation of the shared meal already begins with the shopping trip: "For this meal, I'll first go to the farmers' market, buy some fresh vegetables, and also get flowers for the table..." The cooking process itself can be celebrated with time and love and doesn't have to be relegated to the sidelines. Cooking with fresh and natural foods also increases the sensual experience of the meal as well as our appreciation for the foods and the people who produced them for us. Even though this much effort is not possible on a daily basis, we can still reserve it for special moments. Cooking together with your family or friends can even be a whole lot of fun.

To assist you in your food selection, here is a guidance table for a wholesome, sustainable diet. This table categorizes food products by their level of processing (see pp. 139–141).

Guidance Table for a Wholesome, Sustainable Diet

The criteria for categorizing foods in this table are health aspects as well as ecological and social concerns. Of particular importance are the kind and extent of food processing: increasing levels of processing generally reduces nutrient density while the ecological drawbacks increase. Transitions between columns are sometimes fluid.

As much as possible, choose products from organic agriculture. In addition, we recommend favoring foods that are locally produced and in season. Foods from developing countries, like coffee, tea, and cocoa, should be from Fair Trade. Lastly, avoid any foods that have a particularly high load of harmful residues, as well as foods that contain additives or are enriched with isolated nutrients (with the exception of iodine); also products that were produced through genetic engineering, and unnecessarily packaged foods.

How to Read this Table

Choose foods from the first and second columns each for approximately half of your personal daily amount of food (measured in grams, not calories).[9] Foods from the third column should be consumed only rarely, and column four should be avoided altogether. A star (*) means that you should use these foods in moderation; this quantitative limitation is implied in columns three and four by the title and is therefore not repeated there.

Note: you should give preference to foods that are listed higher up, that is, plant-based ones, over animal-based ones.

Guidance table for a wholesome, sustainable diet—recommendations for food selection for healthy adults[9]

Value Rating	1 Highly Recommended	2 Highly Recommended	3 Less Recommended	4 Not Recommended
Level of processing	Unprocessed/lightly processed foods (unheated)	Moderately processed foods (especially with heat)	Heavily processed foods (especially preserved)	Over-processed foods and isolates/preparations
Recommended amount	Roughly half of your daily food choice	Roughly half of your daily food choice	Consume only rarely	Avoid as much as possible
Vegetables/fruit	Fresh vegetables Lactic acid fermented vegetables (e.g., fresh sauerkraut) Fresh fruit	Heated vegetables (also lactic acid fermented) Heated fruit Frozen fruit and vegetables*	Canned vegetables (e.g., canned tomatoes) Fruit preserves (e.g., cherries in glass jars)	Dietary supplements (e.g., vitamin, mineral, fiber supplements) Frozen ready-made foods

* Use moderately

Guidance table for a wholesome, sustainable diet—recommendations for food selection for healthy adults[9]

Value Rating	1 Highly Recommended	2 Highly Recommended	3 Less Recommended	4 Not Recommended
Level of processing	Unprocessed/lightly processed foods (unheated)	Moderately processed foods (especially with heat)	Heavily processed foods (especially preserved)	Over-processed foods and isolates/preparations
Recommended amount	Roughly half of your daily food choice	Roughly half of your daily food choice	Consume only rarely	Avoid as much as possible
Grain	Sprouted grain Wholegrain meal (e.g., fresh grain muesli) Freshly rolled flakes	Wholegrain products (e.g., wholegrain bread, noodles, flakes, pastries) Wholegrain dishes	Products that are not wholegrain (e.g., white bread, rye bread, white noodles, cornflakes, refined flour pastries) Husked (white) rice	Grain starch (e.g., corn starch)
Potatoes		Cooked potatoes (ideally in the skin)	Ready-made products (e.g., instant mixes for purées or dumplings, potato chips) French fries	Potato starch
Legumes		Sprouted, blanched legumes Heated legumes	Soy milk, tofu Ready-made dishes (e.g., tofu burgers)	Soy "meat" Soy protein Soy lecithin
Nuts/fats/oils	Nuts*, almonds* Oilseeds* (e.g., sunflower seeds, sesame seeds) Oily fruits* (e.g., olives)	Roasted nuts*, nut butters* Native cold-pressed oils* Non-hydrogenated plant margarines—with a high proportion of native cold-pressed oils* Butter*	Salted nuts Extracted, refined fats and oils Non-hydrogenated plant margarines Coconut oil Rendered butter	Nut (chocolate) spreads Hydrogenated fats (e.g., most margarines, deep frying oils) Fat replacements
Milk/dairy products	Certified raw milk	Pasteurized whole milk Dairy products (without additional ingredients) Cheese* (without additives)	UHT milk (products) Dairy products (with additional ingredients) Cheese (with additives)	Sterile milk Condensed milk Powdered milk Lactose Milk and whey protein Milk and cheese imitations Processed cheese

* Use moderately

Guidance table for a wholesome, sustainable diet—recommendations for food selection for healthy adults[9]

Value Rating	1 Highly Recommended	2 Highly Recommended	3 Less Recommended	4 Not Recommended
Level of processing	Unprocessed/lightly processed foods (unheated)	Moderately processed foods (especially with heat)	Heavily processed foods (especially preserved)	Over-processed foods and isolates/preparations
Recommended amount	Roughly half of your daily food choice	Roughly half of your daily food choice	Consume only rarely	Avoid as much as possible
Meat/fish/eggs		Meat* (up to twice/week) Fish* (up to once/week) Eggs* (up to 2/week)	Meat products, fresh or canned Sausage products, fresh or canned Fish products, fresh or canned	Organ meats (except from organically raised animals) Powdered and liquid eggs
Drinks	Unchlorinated drinking water Tested spring water Natural mineral water	Herb and fruit teas* Diluted fruit juices Diluted vegetable juices Grain coffee	Bottled water Fruit nectars Hot chocolate Coffee Black tea Beer, wine	Sodas Fruit juice drinks Instant drinks (e.g., tea, hot chocolate) Sports drinks Energy drinks Other alcoholic drinks
Spices/herbs/salt	Whole or freshly ground spices Fresh herbs	Ground spices Dried herbs Iodized sea salt and table salt*	Herbed salt Sea salt Table salt	Aromas (natural, nature-identical, artificial) Flavor enhancers (e.g., MSG)
Sweeteners	Fresh, sweet fruit	Honey* (not heat-damaged, diluted) Dried fruit* (unsulfured, soaked)	Honey (heat-damaged) Dried fruit (sulfured) Juice concentrates (e.g., from apples, agave) Syrup (e.g., from maple, sugar beets) Unrefined beet sugar Unrefined cane sugar	Confectionery Sweets Isolated sugar (e.g., household sugar and brown sugar) Sugar replacements (e.g., sorbitol) Artificial sweeteners

* Use moderately

"Fair Play" with Foods

Even though we may be upset about price increases, we in the West spend a lower proportion of our income on food in comparison with the past and many other countries: on average only about 13% of the income in France, about 11% in Germany and the Netherlands, about 9% in the UK, and about 7% in the United States.[35]

Measured against our increased income in the West, food expenses have never before been as low as they are today! Many agribusinesses, including farmers, processors, and retailers, however, are no longer able to cover the costs of their operations because of the continuing drop in food-related revenues—whether in industrialized or in so-called developing countries. As a result, more and more agribusinesses have either been going out of business or are forced to operate according to the dictates of their overhead costs—leading to increased problems for sustainability.

Compounding this problem is the fact that the low food prices do not honestly reflect the real costs of production. The resulting ecological and social costs, for example, due to climate damage, pollution in soils and groundwater, or job loss or threat to livelihoods, are not included in the cost of food. The low store prices for food are subsidized by our taxes—or maintained (even more problematically) by transferring follow-up costs to other people, mainly in developing countries, or to future generations. This is the exact opposite of sustaina-

bility—but we can do something about this.

Imported foods from developing countries, like coffee, tea, cocoa/chocolate, tropical fruits, and spices, are a luxury and enrich our everyday lives. Only a few people are aware, however, where exactly these goods come from and how they were produced in the countries of the "Global South." Many agricultural products and consumer items are manufactured under inhumane working conditions, often by children. Eighty million, or 40% of all children under 14 in Africa, for example, are affected by exploitative forms of child labor.[36] They are suffering under forced labor, bondage, slavery, or abuse. They are not able to go to school, and most of them do not receive any wages.

We can support sustainable and therefore socially acceptable development in the developing countries if we are willing to pay fair prices for imported goods. Certified goods from Fair Trade are offered in so-called world markets or in health food stores, and by now even in many supermarkets. When we purchase local

products directly from the producer, we can even ask personally whether the price really adds up.

Does the Price Add Up?

Local farmers also need fair and stable prices that cover their costs. For most dairy farmers in Germany, for example, the costs associated with the production of milk are higher than the profit they can currently get on the market. A liter of milk often costs only about half as much as a liter of gasoline—and little of that actually goes back to the dairy farmer. While production costs mostly increase steadily, the producer price for milk is marked by continuous fluctuations. In the beginning of 2008, for example, it was 40 cents per liter in Bavaria; in July 2009, however, it was only 24 cents and in the spring of 2011, it had risen back up to 33 cents.[37]

Global prices for conventionally traded imported products from developing countries fluctuate greatly as well. In the global Fair Trade network, however, producers receive a fair minimum price for raw materials like coffee or cocoa beans that is higher than the price on the world market and covers the costs of production. Even better, premiums and commitments to purchase are specified in long-term contracts, which provide the farmers with security for planning. And advance payments through the importers make important investments possible. With Fair Trade foods the intermediary broker is eliminated through direct purchase. In contrast, a large portion of the sale price in conventional products ends up with the brokers. For farmers, direct purchase of their products thus secures a considerably higher price.[38]

Why We Should Pay Fair Producer Prices

When we pay fair producer prices for domestic products we support smaller and medium-sized operations. This secures jobs in rural areas. These agricultural operations in addition help to maintain the cultural landscape, including the animals, for example mountainside pasture management in alpine areas or flocks of sheep in heathland areas.

Because producers of Fair Trade goods in developing countries are for the most part democratically organized farmers' associations, they can then decide on their own how to spend their extra income—social projects, advanced training, health care, and infrastructure.[38] Fair Trade actively supports the creation of social institutions like schools, hospitals, or retirement homes, and guarantees social security for farmers and laborers. In addition, Fair Trade strengthens the qualifications and self-confidence of producers —and explicitly eliminates exploitative forms of child labor.[36]

As long as it is not clear, however, why conventional foods are so cheap and Fair Trade products more expensive, they are more likely to get left behind on store shelves. Public education and awareness-building are therefore necessary to make the higher price of Fair Trade products from developing countries transparent and to motivate consumers to purchase them. These efforts must also be financed through the higher price of the products.

Fair Mainly Also Means Organic

The conditions of production in Fair Trade include minimum environmental safety requirements like protection of the drinking water, reforestation, waste removal, and the minimization of chemical applications. Products from Fair Trade are now mainly produced with certified organic quality and are therefore subject to even stricter environmental regulations.

FACTS

Fluctuations in the Price of Coffee and Their Effects

Here is an example of how much prices for certain agricultural products fluctuate on the world market. In 2008, 500 g Arabica coffee brought an average of €0.87 in conventional trade; in 2001, for example, it only brought €0.46. The guaranteed price for Fair Trade coffee was at least €0.93 in 2008, in addition to a Fair Trade premium of €0.07—thus a total of at least €1. This price was negotiated between the Fair Trade organizations and the producers—and at least secured a minimum subsistence level for the families of laborers and farmers.[38] In the middle of 2011, however, the price for Arabica coffee on the world market was at €2.15 per 500 g, or roughly twice as high as in 2008. The reasons for this considerable increase were unusually difficult harvest and transport conditions due to bad weather, as well as stock market speculations and an increase in demand especially in the emerging nations. The price increase on the world market means higher profits for all coffee farmers, while the members of Fair Trade associations additionally receive their special premium. Even though this improves the lives of all coffee farmers, a truly secure livelihood is in the long run guaranteed only with Fair Trade. This fact is demonstrated clearly in the example of October 2001 when coffee prices collapsed completely from one day to the next.

Health Protection for Farmers in Developing Countries

Enhanced health and safety measures, for example, wearing protective suits for the application of chemical substances, allow farmers and laborers in developing countries to avoid poisoning and other health problems. Their higher income in Fair Trade gives producers more money for food and education, which contributes to better nutrition and health.

Coffee, tea, cocoa, and chocolate offer us a conscious pleasure. To enjoy them in moderation benefits our health and balances out the higher price we pay for Fair Trade products. Fair Trade foods are recognizable by specific logos (see illustrations).

Examples of Logos for Products from Fair Trade

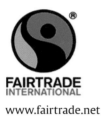

FAIRTRADE
INTERNATIONAL
www.fairtrade.net

www.fairtradeusa.org

www.rainforest-alliance.org

www.twin.org.uk

www.wfto.com

www.fairforlife.net

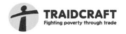
www.traidcraft.co.uk

www.equal-exchange.coop

www.fta.org.au

FACTS

Campaigns for Fair Trade

A number of related organizations conduct educational and advocacy campaigns with reference to Fair Trade objectives, suppliers, and producers.

The "Fair Trade Towns" campaign, for instance, is a dynamic global movement of cities and communities who are helping to grow Fair Trade. There are now 1136 Fair Trade Towns on five continents, which makes this the biggest campaign promoting Fair Trade worldwide (www.fairtradetowns.org). In 2012, among other topics, the program included the launch of the international campaign "United Nations Post-2015 Millennium Development Goals" (www.un.org/millenniumgoals). These have been supplemented as a result of the Rio+20 Conference by the United Nations Sustainable Development Goals (www.sustainabledevelopment.un.org).

Another example of campaigning to advance Fair Trade objectives is World Food Day, organized by The Food and Agriculture Organization of the United Nations (FAO) and observed annually on 16 October since 1979 by many thousands of organizations and individuals across the world (www.fao.org/getinvolved/worldfoodday/en).

The fact that Fair Trade and ecological agriculture can make a significant contribution to global food security was confirmed by the report, **Agriculture at a Crossroads,** published by the International Assessment of Agricultural Knowledge, Science and Technology for Development (IAASTD) in 2008 (www.agassessment.org).

Sustainability in Everyday Life

"Sort your trash," "Avoid packaging"—such advice has made some inroads with consumers. But what about avoiding trash altogether? How can we save electricity? And what should we pay attention to when purchasing household appliances or during shopping trips?

Packaging Waste and Trash

As a matter of fact, Germany and other countries of Northern Europe are ahead of the rest of the world when it comes to sorting trash. Avoiding trash altogether, however, is an area where much work remains to be done. It is necessary to do so in order to reduce our mountains of trash over the long run, for example when we think of the amount of plastic bags consumed each year per person. Plastic bags are not biodegradable and do not decompose.

When we properly separate plastic bags from regular household trash and dispose of them in the recycling bin, they can be processed into recycled plastic. Another portion ends up in our end waste, which in most cases is burned, potentially producing substances that are toxic and harmful to the climate. In addition, innumerable bags make their way into nature without getting properly disposed of at all. These gradually break apart into smaller and smaller pieces, stressing the environment and endangering many animals.

While disposable plastic bags are still everywhere in the United States, many cities (for example, Portland) now have ordinances that ban the use of disposable plastic bags. Also, large chain stores like Wal-Mart or Target do now collect used plastic bags for recycling. And in Hong Kong an environmental levy of 50 cents on each plastic shopping bag has been proposed.[39]

What Can We Do?
- To avoid trash, buy your food as much as possible unpackaged, for example, vegetables, potatoes, and fruit. Alternatively, choose foods that come in reusable packaging. As a rule, these are better for the environment than those in disposable packages, let alone minimum-sized containers. Please feel free to leave multiple-packaged products on the shelf.
- Before you go shopping, always remember to bring along appropriate bags and containers, and reuse them as often as possible. In this way you can always avoid new plastic bags.
- Also, do give less than perfectly grown vegetables and fruits a

---

FACTS

Food Turns into Trash

In the United States, for example, nearly 50% of all food becomes trash.[40] Food scraps, products with recently expired "best before" dates, and fruits and vegetables with minor blemishes are thrown out, to say nothing of the huge amounts of food that supermarkets or the food service industry dispose of on a large scale. Many cities have, on the other hand, begun to set up places where stores and restaurants can deposit their excess food, to have it distributed to people in need.

chance, not only standardized blemish-free produce.
- Are you leaving for a trip and have food left in the fridge that you can't take with you? Give it away to friends and neighbors so that these treats don't spoil.
- If you can't finish your meal in a restaurant, you can take the leftovers home in a box.

Switching to Green Energy: The Key to Climate Protection

Even if we have internalized tips for saving electricity in the household and use energy-efficient appliances it is impossible to reduce our energy consumption to zero. Nevertheless, if you switch your energy provider and purchase green energy from renewable sources, you can reduce the harmful effect of your energy consumption substantially (about 90%).

The current composition of energy sources for producing electricity varies all over the world. The situation is complex in Canada and the United States as the provinces and states generally generate their own power locally. For example, some provinces in Canada, like Quebec and Manitoba, have almost 100% hydroelectricity, while others, like Saskatchewan and Alberta, have closer to 60–70% coal. There is some exchange across borders (including the Canada–United States border), but by and large most provinces consume what they produce.[41]

On a national scale, most of the electricity in the United States—as per statistics from the US Energy Information Administration, 2011—is produced using steam turbines, which are powered by coal (42%), natural gas (25%), nuclear power (19%), hydropower (8%), wind power (3%), and petroleum, biomass, geothermal power, and solar power (each at less than 1%).[41]

In comparison, the electricity mix in the United Kingdom—figures from 2011 supplied by the Department of Energy and Climate Change (DECC)—shows the following picture by fuel type: natural gas (41%), coal (29%), nuclear power (18%), hydropower and other fuels (5%), wind power (4%), and oil (1%).[42]

The nuclear disaster in Japan in 2011 has taught us once again in a dramatic fashion that atomic energy is not a safe alternative to electricity from fossil fuel sources like coal, oil, or gas. Thus, the following combination of measures represents the only sensible alternative:

- Increasing the technological efficiency of electricity usage
- Consistent and comprehensive energy conservation (sufficiency) in all areas of life and society
- Generation of the electricity that we require from renewable sources like water, wind, sun, and geothermal sources

The United Nations has established the global initiative, "Sustainable Energy for All," with similar goals in mind. The aim of the initiative is to mobilize all sectors of society worldwide in support of three interlinked objectives to be achieved by 2030: providing universal access to modern energy services, doubling the global rate of improvement in energy efficiency, and doubling the share of renewable energy in the global energy mix. In conjunction with this ambitious project, the UN has declared 2012 the "International Year of Sustainable Energy for All." For information on both programs, please see www.sustainableenergyforall.org.

Switching to a green energy provider is very easy and quick, with no loss of convenience, in many cases not more expensive—and a clear political signal for the necessary energy turnaround. Further information on finding a suitable green energy provider can be found, for example, here: www.renewableenergyworld.com/rea/partner/search.

Saving Energy in the Kitchen

Even if you have already made the switch to green energy it also has to be generated and transported and the equipment must be built. Therefore, a small burden on the climate remains, approximately 10% of the previous energy. In addition, the generation of energy is cost-intensive. It is therefore worth saving energy—for the climate and for the wallet.

When Cooking and Baking[43]

- Choose a burner or hot plate that is appropriate for the size of the bottom of the pot, because otherwise you waste a lot of energy.
- If you want to avoid wasting around 75% of the energy used in cooking and losing important ingredients from your food through evaporation, use lids that fit your pots and pans. Glass lids are best because you don't have to lift them so often to check the food inside. Cook with as little liquid as possible.
- Take advantage of the residual heat produced by stove burners or hot plates by turning them off earlier.
- When you need hot water to make tea or coffee or cook noodles or potatoes, it is best to heat it in an electric water kettle.
- If possible, don't preheat the oven before baking but take advantage of the convection function, if applicable, and of residual heat after you turn the oven off. You can also cook several dishes or parts of dishes at the same time.

- As much as possible, cook or bake larger amounts at a time—also for the next day.

When Cooling and Freezing[44]

- Organize your food neatly in the fridge and freezer so that you don't have to keep the door open as long to find something, otherwise too much cold escapes.
- For fresh food and reduced energy consumption, you shouldn't keep your refrigerator colder than 7–8 °C. A modern freshness drawer, set at ca. 1 °C, is ideal for crunchy vegetables and fruit. And if you eat your vegetables and fruit quickly, things like apples or tomatoes don't need to go into the fridge at all. A cool basement is often enough for several days.
- As a rule of thumb, freezing requires a large amount of electricity, especially for ensuring an unbroken cold chain in retail. For our daily diet, frozen products therefore don't make much sense in ecological terms but should rather be used for special or unexpected occasions. Freezing may also be an option for winter when not many fresh fruits and vegetables are available from local sources, as well as for storing produce from your own garden.
- If you want to preserve leftovers from a meal, let them cool down first before putting them in the fridge or freezer.

- Thick layers of ice greatly increase electricity consumption. It is therefore important to defrost your cooling appliances regularly.
- Defrosting frozen foods is best done in the refrigerator, which as a result doesn't have to start up again so quickly and thus consumes less electricity.

When Washing Dishes[44]

- Dishwashers generally use less water and energy than if you were to wash the same amount of dishes by hand.
- Take advantage of energy-saving settings and turn the machine off as soon as the program is finished.
- Avoid unnecessary pre-rinsing of dishes.
- Use your detergent sparingly and only turn the dishwasher on when it is full.

Energy-efficient Household Appliances

Large electrical appliances like refrigerators, dishwashers, and washing machines can be real energy hogs. In the United States we can recognize appliances that consume less energy by energy guide labels: these compare the usage for different models, give us the estimated yearly operating cost, as well as the estimated yearly electricity usage. In the EU, there are labels that range from A++ for highly efficient to G for highly inefficient. A washing machine or dishwasher that consumes relatively small amounts of energy, for example, is marked with

133

the best energy efficiency rating A. In refrigerators and freezers, the rating A++ marks the best appliances. Even if these can be more expensive to purchase initially, it pays off over their service lifetime.

Over time, a lot of small electrical appliances accumulate in the kitchen. The average Western industrialized household owns between 10 and 15 such devices: electric knives, can openers, ice crushers, hotplates, toasters, or juicers. But do we really need all these little electro-helpers? And if so, how often? Maybe a little manual labor and therefore more exercise would even be good for us?

TIP

Shopping Help with Regard to Energy Criteria

In addition to selected household appliances, the website www.energystar.gov also includes information on building products and on heating and cooling. Energy Star is a joint program of the US Environmental Protection Agency and the US Department of Energy to label products that help save money and protect the environment through energy-efficient products and practices. Earning the Energy Star means products meet strict energy efficiency guidelines set by the US Environmental Protection Agency.

Shopping Trips: Better on Foot or by Bike

For our grocery shopping trips, cars are the most environmentally harmful mode of transportation. Especially for only short distances, the car is the worst choice possible because a cold engine uses more gasoline for the first mile.[45] If we regularly use the car to go grocery shopping this can offset, for example, all our efforts that we have made to achieve a climate-friendly diet by reducing animal products and purchasing more ecological foods and local and seasonal products.

By walking or switching to the bicycle, public transportation, or car pools, you protect the climate—and your wallet. On shorter trips, you are better off on foot anyway and reach your destination more quickly than by driving (including the time for walking to and from the car, opening and closing doors, getting in and out of the car, looking for a parking spot, parking, etc.).[45]

Even better, walking or cycling offers healthy exercise in fresh air. Cycling is refreshing: when we cycle to work, we are more awake and productive when we get there. In addition, we can lower the risk of excess weight, cardiovascular disorders, and type 2 diabetes.

References

1 von Koerber K, Kretschmer J. Ernährung nach den vier Dimensionen. Ernährung und Medizin. 2006; 21: 178–185. Available at www.bfeoe.de/EuM-2006-178_185.pdf. Accessed December 29, 2012

2 von Koerber K, Männle T, Leitzmann C. Vollwert-Ernährung—Konzeption einer zeitgemäßen und nachhaltigen Ernährung. Stuttgart: Haug; 2012

3 Food and Agriculture Organization of the United Nations (FAO). Cereals; 2009. Available at www.fao.org/docrep/011/ai482e/ai482e02.htm. Accessed August 10, 2012

4 Bradford E, Baldwin RL, Blackburn H, et al. Animal agriculture and global food supply. Task Force Report No. 135. Ames, Iowa: Council for Agricultural Science and Technology; 1999

5 Food and Agriculture Organization of the United Nations (FAO). Hunger; 2012. Available at www.fao.org/hunger/en/ Accessed December 7, 2012

6 UNICEF. Levels and trends in child mortality; 2011. Available at www.unicef.org/media/files/Child_Mortality_Report_2011_Final.pdf. Accessed December 12, 2011

7 Keller M. Flugimporte von Lebensmitteln und Blumen nach Deutschland. Eine Untersuchung im Auftrag der Verbraucherzentrale. Frankfurt/M: Verbraucherzentrale Hessen; 2010. Available at www.vzhh.de/docs/100187/Studie%20Flugimporte_Deutschland%202010.pdf. Accessed December 29, 2012

8 U.S. Department of Agriculture and U.S. Department of Health and Human Services. Dietary Guidelines for Americans. Appendices 8 and 9 (Vegetarian Adaptations). 7th ed. Washington, DC: U.S. Government Printing Office; 2010. Available at www.dietaryguidelines.gov. Accessed December 31, 2012

9 Männle T, von Koerber K, Leitzmann C, Hoffmann I, von Hollen A, Franz W. Orientierungstabelle für die Vollwert-Ernährung—Empfehlungen für die Lebensmittelauswahl gesunder Erwachsender. Verbraucher-Zentrale NRW und Verband für Unabhängige Gesundheitsberatung – Deutschland (Hrsg.), UGB-Beratungs- und Verlags-GmbH; 2000

10 Food and Agriculture Organization of the United Nations (FAO). Livestock and fish primary equivalent, 02 June 2010. FAOSTAT online statistical service. Rome: FAO; 2010. Available at knoema.com/UNFAOFSSLSF2010Jun. Accessed January 8, 2013

11 International Energy Agency. Selected 2009 indicators for the United States. Available at www.iea.org/stats/indicators.asp?COUNTRY_CODE=US. Accessed August 10, 2012. Selected 2009 indicators for European Union. Available at www.iea.org/stats/indicators.asp?COUNTRY_CODE=30. Accessed August 10, 2012

12 International Energy Agency. World energy outlook 2011. Available at www.worldenergyoutlook.org/publications/weo-2011/. Accessed January 8, 2013

13 Food and Agriculture Organization of the United Nations (FAO). Livestock's long shadow. Environmental issues and options. Rome: FAO; 2006. Available at www.fao.org/docrep/010/a0701e/a0701e00.HTM. Accessed August 10, 2010

14 Mekonnen MM, Hoekstra AY. The green, blue and grey water footprint of crops and derived crop products. Hydrology and Earth System Sciences. 2011;15: 1577–1600

15 Mekonnen MM, Hoekstra AY. A global assessment of the water footprint of farm animal products. Ecosystems 2012;15:401–415

16 Peters CJ, Wilkins JL, Fick GW. Testing a complete-diet model for estimating the land resource requirements of food consumption and agricultural carrying capacity—the New York State example. Renewable Agriculture and Food Systems 2007;22:145–153

17 Food and Agriculture Organization, Statistics Division (FAOSTAT). Data archives; 2008. Available at www.faostat.fao.org. Accessed March 20, 2008

18 Idel A. Die Kuh ist kein Klima-Killer! Wie die Agrarindustrie die Erde verwüstet und was wir dagegen tun können. Marburg: Metropolis; 2010

19 Food and Agriculture Organization Statistics Division (FAOSTAT). Data by domain; 2010. Available at faostat3.fao.org/home/index.html#VISUALIZE_BY_DOMAIN. Accessed August 10, 2012

20 Food and Agriculture Organization of the United Nations (FAO). Are grasslands under threat?; 2008. Available at www.fao.org/ag/agp/agpc/doc/grass_stats/grass-stats.htm. Accessed August 10, 2012

21 Leitzmann C, Keller M. Vegetarische Ernährung. Stuttgart: Eugen Ulmer; 2010

22 Pimentel D. Impacts of organic farming on the efficiency of energy use in agriculture. Organic Center State of Science Review. Cornell University; 2006. Available at www.organic-center.org under "State of Science Review". Accessed August 13, 2012

23 Badgley C, Moghtader J, Quintero E, et al. Organic agriculture and the global food supply. Renewable Agriculture and Food Systems 2007;22:86–108

24 Bockisch FJ (Ed.). Bewertung von Verfahren der ökologischen und konventionellen landwirtschaftlichen Produktion im Hinblick auf den Energieeinsatz und bestimmte Schadgasemissionen. Braunschweig: Bundesforschungsanstalt für Landwirtschaft; 2000

25 Hörtenhuber S, Zollitsch W. Treibhausgase von der Weide. Welche Vorteile bringt die Öko-Rinderhaltung? Ökologie und Landbau 2008;36(1):23–25

26 Pimentel D. Soil erosion: a food and environmental threat. Environment, Development and Sustainability 2006;8:119–137

27 International Assessment of Agricultural Knowledge, Science and Technology for Development (IAASTD). Agriculture at a crossroads: the global report. Washington, DC: Island Press; 2009

28 Benbrook C, Zhao X, Yáñez J, Davies J, Andrews P. New evidence confirms the nutritional superiority of plant-based organic foods. Organic Center State of Science Review. Cornell University; 2008. Available at www.organic-center. org under "State of Science Review." Accessed August 14, 2012

29 Cross P, Edwards RT, Hounsome B, Edward-Jones G. Comparative assessment of migrant farm worker health in conventional and organic horticultural systems in the United Kingdom. Science of the Total Environment 2008;391:55–65

30 Ho MW, Gala R. Food miles and sustainability. What's behind the statistics and what should be done? ISIS Report; 2005. Available at www.i-sis.org.uk/FMAS. php. Accessed January 8, 2013

31 Garnett T. Fruit and vegetables & UK greenhouse gas emissions: exploring the relationship. Working paper 06-01 Rev. A; 2006. Available at www.fcrn.org. uk/sites/default/files/fruitveg_paper_ final.pdf. Accessed January 8, 2013

32 Elmadfa I, Aign W, Muskat E, Fritzsche D. Die große GU Nährwert-Kalorien-Tabelle. München: Gräfe und Unzer; 2009

33 Hoffmann I. Ernährungsempfehlungen und Ernährungsweisen – Auswirkungen auf Gesundheit, Umwelt und Gesellschaft. Habilitationsschrift, Fachbereich Agrarwissenschaften, Ökotrophologie und Umweltmanagement der Universität Gießen; 2002

34 Öko-Institut e.V. Datenbank GEMIS – Globales Emissions-Modell integrierter Systeme, Version 4.5; 2009. Available at www.gemis.de. Accessed October 27, 2009

35 Sorensen E. Billions served. Washington State Magazine 2001;Fall:39–45. Available at wsm.wsu.edu/researcher/ 2011fall_hunger_foodcost.php. Accessed January 9, 2013

36 International Labour Organization (ILO). About child labour; 2009. Available at www.ilo.org. Accessed October 27, 2009

37 Bayerische Landesanstalt für Landwirtschaft – Institut für Ernährung und Markt: aktuell–Monatsstatistiken; 2011. Available at www.lfl.bayern.de/ iem/milchwirtschaft/06935/index.php. Accessed April 29, 2011

38 Fairtrade International. Aims of fairtrade standards; 2011. Available at www.fairtrade.net/aims_of_fairtrade_standards. html. Accessed October 11, 2012

39 Environmental levy on plastic shopping bags; 2 February 2011. Available at www.epd.gov.hk/epd/english/environ mentinhk/waste/prob_solutions/env_ levy.html. Accessed January 10, 2013

40 Jonathan Bloom. American wasteland: how America throws away nearly half of its food (and what we can do about it). Cambridge, MA: Da Capo Lifelong Books; 2010

41 U.S. Energy Information Administration. Monthly Energy Review (March 2012). Available at www.eia.gov/energyexplained. Accessed January 10, 2013

42 UK Guide to National and Official Statistics. Available at www.gov.uk/government/organisations/department-of-energy-climate-change. Accessed March 18, 2013

43 Öko-Institut. Fragen und Antworten zum Kochen und Backen; 2009. Available at www.ecotopten.de/prod_ kochen_faq.php. Accessed March 2, 2011

44 Stadtwerke München. Energietipps; 2006. Available at www.swm.de/dms/ swm/dokumente/kundenservice/ energieberatung/energiespar-tipps.pdf. Accessed March 2, 2011

45 Verkehrsclub Deutschland (VCD). CO2-Einsparpotentiale; 2010. Available at www.vcd.org/einsparpotenziale.html. Mobil mit dem Auto; 2010. Available at www.vcd.org/1064.html. Mobil zu Fuß und mit dem Rad; 2011. Available at www.vcd.org/1068.html, 2011. All accessed March 2, 2011

Further Links

Here is a list of useful further links. Of the vast amount of available sources, this is only a selection to give the reader guidance to further research on the topics of the book.

Sustainability

www.unesco.org/new/en/education/themes/leading-the-international-agenda/education-for-sustainable-development (UNESCO, Education for Sustainable Development)
www.desd.org (UN Decade of Education for Sustainable Development)
www.rce-network.org/elgg (Regional Centers of Expertise on Education for Sustainable Development)
www.millennium-institute.org (Millennium Institute)
www.oekosozial.at (Eco Social Forum)
www.globalmarshallplan.org/en (Global Marshall Plan Initiative)

Healthy/Sustainable Nutrition

www.iuns.org (International Union of Nutritional Sciences)
www.slowfood.com (Slow Food International)
www.terramadre.org (Terra Madre Organization)
www.vrg.org (The Vegetarian Resource Group, USA)
www.vegsoc.org (Vegetarian Society, UK)
www.buchinger.com/en/welcome-to-buchinger.html (Buchinger Clinic, English language site)
www.ne.wzw.tum.de (Working Group Sustainable Nutrition, Technische Universität München, Germany)

Environment/Climate

www.unep.org (United Nations Environment Programme)

www.thinkeatsave.org (Think.Eat.Save Campaign)
www.ipcc.ch (Intergovernmental Panel on Climate Change)
http://unfccc.int (UN Framework Convention on Climate Change)
www.greenpeace.org/international/en (Greenpeace International)
www.worldwildlife.org (World Wildlife Fund)
www.thefern.org (Food and Environment Reporting Network)
http://co2now.org (CO2 Now Organization)
www.pear-energy.com (Pear Energy, USA, Green Energy)
www.sustainableenergyforall.org (Sustainable Energy for All)

Organic Agriculture

www.soilassociation.org (Soil Association)
www.ams.usda.gov/nop (National Organic Program, USA)
www.ota.com (Organic Trade Association, USA)
www.farmers.coop (Cooperative Regions of Organic Producer Pools, USA)
www.biodynamics.com (Biodynamic Farming and Gardening Association)
www.hfa.org (The Humane Farming Association, USA)
www.gardenorganic.org.uk (Garden Organic, UK)

Regional/Local Foods

www.localharvest.org (Local Harvest Organization, UK)
www.beneficialfarm.com (Beneficial Farm CSA, USA)
www.sappingtonfarmersmkt.com (Farm to Family Naturally, LLC, USA)
www.gorgegrown.com (Gorge Grown Food Network, USA)
www.greenbeandelivery.com (Green B.E.A.N. Delivery, USA)

www.tusimbolo.org (Foundation of Organized Small Producers, Latin America)

World Nutrition

www.fao.org (Food and Agriculture Organization of the United Nations)
www.who.int/nutrition/topics/nutrecomm/en/index.html (WHO Dietary Recommendation, Nutritional Requirements)
www.agassessment.org (Agricultural Knowledge, Science and Technology for Development, IAASTD)
www.ifpri.cgiar.org (International Food Policy Research Institute)
www.fian.org (Food First Information and Action Network)
www.wholeplanetfoundation.org (Whole Planet Foundation)

Fair Trade

www.fairtrade.net (Fairtrade International)
www.fairtradeusa.org (Fair Trade USA)
www.fairtrade.org.uk (Fairtrade Foundation, UK)
www.fta.org.au (Fair Trade Australia New Zealand)
www.fairtradeafrica.net (Fairtrade Africa)
www.wfto.com (World Fair Trade Organization)
www.equalexchange.coop (Equal Exchange)
www.fairtradetowns.org (Fair Trade Towns)
www.gepa.de/p/index.php/mID/1/lan/en (GEPA, European Fair Trade)
www.terredeshommes.org (Terre des Hommes, International Federation)

Index of Recipes

Subject Index